360.

geriatrics

The National Medical Series for Independent Study

geriatrics

EDITORS

Douglas C. Conaway, M.D.

Assistant Professor of Medicine
Rheumatology Section
Temple University School of Medicine
Attending Physician
Temple University Hospital
Philadelphia, Pennsylvania

Max D. Miller, Ed.D.

Professor of Family Medicine
Associate Director, Ambulatory Geriatric Care Program
Medical College of Georgia
Augusta, Georgia

Glenn R. West, Ph.D.

Assistant Professor of Continuing Education and Health Communication
Medical College of Georgia
Augusta, Georgia

A WILEY MEDICAL PUBLICATION
JOHN WILEY & SONS
New York • Chichester • Brisbane • Toronto • Singapore

Harwal Publishing Company, Media, Pennsylvania

Library of Congress Cataloging in Publication Data
Main entry under title:

Geriatrics.

(The National medical series for independent study. Exam series) (A Wiley medical publication)
1. Geriatrics—Examinations, questions, etc.
I. Conaway, Douglas C., 1950- . II. West, Glenn R.
III. Miller, Max D., 1940- IV. Series.
V. Series: Wiley medical publication.
RC952.6.G47 1988 618.97′0076 88-117
ISBN 0-471-61373-8 (pbk.)

10 9 8 7 6 5 4 3 2 1

Contents

Contributors

Robert J. Adams, M.D.
Assistant Professor of Neurology
Medical College of Georgia
Attending Physician and Neurological Consultant
Veterans Administration Medical Center
Augusta, Georgia

Reid B. Blackwelder, M.D.
Instructor of Family Medicine
Medical College of Georgia
Augusta, Georgia

William G. Caput, M.D., M.P.H., M.H.A.
Associate Professor of Family Medicine
Vice Chairman and Director, Family Practice Center
Medical College of Georgia
Augusta, Georgia

Douglas C. Conaway, M.D.
Assistant Professor of Medicine
Rheumatology Section
Temple University School of Medicine
Attending Physician
Temple University Hospital
Philadelphia, Pennsylvania

Mary Ann Forney, Ph.D.
Assistant Professor of Family Medicine
Medical College of Georgia
Augusta, Georgia

Paul D. Forney, M.D.
Associate Professor of Family Medicine
Medical College of Georgia
Augusta, Georgia

R. Leon Longe, Pharm.D.
Associate Professor of Clinical Pharmacy
College of Pharmacy
University of Georgia
Athens, Georgia
Associate Clinical Professor of Family Medicine
Medical College of Georgia
Augusta, Georgia

Max D. Miller, Ed.D.
Professor of Family Medicine
Associate Director, Ambulatory Geriatric Care Program
Medical College of Georgia
Augusta, Georgia

George A. Nixon, M.D.
Assistant Professor of Family Medicine
Medical College of Georgia
Augusta, Georgia

K. D. Sethi, M.D., M.R.C.P. (U.K.)
Assistant Professor of Neurology
Medical College of Georgia
Augusta, Georgia

A. Thomas Taylor, Pharm.D.
Associate Professor of Clinical Pharmacy
College of Pharmacy
University of Georgia
Athens, Georgia
Associate Clinical Professor of Family Medicine
Medical College of Georgia
Augusta, Georgia

Samuel B. Thielman, M.D., Ph.D.
Assistant Professor of Psychiatry
Head of Geriatrics Section
Medical College of Georgia
Augusta, Georgia

Mason P. Thompson, M.D.
Associate Professor of Family Medicine
Medical College of Georgia
Augusta, Georgia

Jay R. Varma, M.D.
Assistant Professor of Family Medicine
Medical College of Georgia
Augusta, Georgia

Glenn R. West, Ph.D.
Assistant Professor of Continuing Education and Health Communication
Continuing Education Program Development Coordinator for Ambulatory Geriatrics
Medical College of Georgia
Augusta, Georgia

Preface

Internists, family physicians, and other medical practitioners often evolve into geriatricians without being aware of the evolution. According to patient demographic studies, the mean age of patients being treated by physicians is increasing. Indeed, more time is devoted to the care of elderly patients than is spent caring for any other patient group. For the physician encountering an increasing number of geriatric patients, there is the added responsibility of recognizing and properly managing health problems that are somewhat different from those experienced by younger patients.

The subtle changes that have been occurring at the level of the individual medical practice are beginning to affect national health care policy. A growing percentage of the health care dollar is being spent either by or on behalf of elderly patients. Health care policymakers in the United States are studying the health planning problems being faced by other countries whose populations are older than our own. As the population in this country ages and as medical science further extends the lifespan, these problems are likely to become our problems.

The National Center for Health Statistics has estimated that by the year 2000, the population of the United States will consist of approximately 6.7 million people who are 85 years of age or older. Already, the 75 years and older group is the fastest growing segment of the population. As more people live longer, a greater demand will be placed on the health care system, not only for additional funding to accommodate the wider range and chronicity of medical problems of the elderly, but also for medical providers trained to deal with these problems.

The American Board of Internal Medicine (ABIM) and the American Board of Family Practice (ABFP) have recognized the critical importance of preparing physicians for this future. To that end, the ABIM and ABFP have jointly prepared an examination leading to a Certificate of Added Qualifications in Geriatric Medicine.

The purposes of this book are to provide the physician with an overview of geriatric medicine and to assist him or her in preparing for the ABIM/ABFP examination. These objectives have been met through the careful development of review questions that are pertinent to the general areas covered by the examination and that are presented in the format used in previous ABIM and ABFP examinations.

The Editors

Acknowledgments

The editors find it appropriate to acknowledge the efforts of Debra Dreger, the test development editor at Harwal/Wiley Medical. Her fund of medical knowledge and many hours of careful research and writing have contributed greatly to the creation of this book. The editors also wish to acknowledge Jim Harris, the president of Harwal/Wiley Medical, for recognizing the need for such a book and for his guidance in its creation. Finally, the editorial contributions of Jane Velker also are greatly appreciated as are the enthusiasm and pride that the entire Harwal/Wiley Medical staff has infused into this project.

Introduction

NMS™ *Geriatrics* has been developed chiefly for internists and family practitioners who want to prepare for the certification examination in geriatric medicine that is being given jointly by the American Board of Internal Medicine (ABIM) and the American Board of Family Practice (ABFP). This book also should serve as a useful educational tool for physicians who choose to stay abreast of the advances in medical information concerning the geriatric patient.

The basic components of *Geriatrics* include more than 500 multiple-choice questions, the correct answers, and detailed explanations of the topics covered in the questions. The questions and explanations have been developed with the intent of providing a broad base of knowledge in geriatric medicine and are grouped into 10 chapters that address important areas of this discipline. The overall format of the questions in *Geriatrics* simulates that used in recent certification examinations given by the ABIM, including clinical case management problems.

Each chapter is divided into a section of questions and a section of answers and explanations. The questions are of two types:

1. **Single best answer**. This type consists of a question or an incomplete statement followed by five answers or completions (options). The options always are lettered A, B, C, D, and E. The reader is asked to select the best answer to the question; although other options may be partially correct, there is only one answer.
2. **Multiple true-false**. This type consists of an introductory premise followed by four statements that pertain to the information stated in the premise. The reader is asked to indicate whether each of the statements is true or false.

The answers and explanations at the end of each chapter are intended to provide immediate reinforcement of the knowledge tested in the questions. The explanations have been prepared by the editors and contributing authors on the basis of information contained in the various sources listed in the bibliography that appears at the end of the book. Considerable effort has been made to assure that these discussions are accurate and pertinent to the physician who seeks a clear understanding of the salient issues in geriatric medicine. A glossary also is provided, which includes commonly abbreviated terms that appear in the questions and explanations contained in *Geriatrics*.

1
Clinical Pharmacology

QUESTIONS

Directions: Each question below contains five suggested answers. Choose the **one best** response to each question.

1. Aging is associated with physiologic changes that significantly affect the way geriatric patients respond to potent pharmacologic agents. Such physiologic factors include all of the following EXCEPT

(A) decreased renal function
(B) decreased liver mass
(C) decreased liver enzyme activity
(D) decreased cardiac output
(E) decreased proportion of fat to muscle

2. Reflux esophagitis is a frequent problem in the geriatric age-group, with the primary cause being decreased LES pressure. Drugs known to decrease LES pressure include all of the following EXCEPT

(A) diphenhydramine
(B) theophylline
(C) nitroglycerin
(D) bethanechol
(E) morphine

3. A 74-year-old man complains that he has been having trouble urinating. Which of the following drugs most likely is causing his urinary retention?

(A) Inhaled ipratropium
(B) Oral buspirone
(C) Oral glyburide
(D) Oral hydroxyzine
(E) Ophthalmic timolol

4. Chronic treatment of angina pectoris in a geriatric patient with a history of congestive heart failure and hypertension is best initiated with which of the following medications?

(A) Propranolol
(B) Nifedipine
(C) Metoprolol
(D) Verapamil
(E) Nadolol

5. A 65-year-old man with a 15-year history of hypertension complains that since his last office visit, 3 weeks earlier, he has experienced shortness of breath and fatigue; otherwise, he denies new cardiac complaints. At his last visit, the following alterations were made in his antihypertensive regimen: an increase in propranolol from 40 mg to 80 mg 4 times daily, an increase in hydralazine from 25 mg twice daily to 25 mg 4 times daily, the addition of hydrochlorothiazide 25 mg once daily, and the discontinuation of clonidine 0.1 mg 3 times daily. At today's visit, the patient's blood pressure is 120/70 mm Hg and his pulse is 58/min. What is the most likely cause of this patient's recent complaints?

(A) The increase in the propranolol dosage
(B) The increase in the hydralazine dosage
(C) The addition of hydrochlorothiazide
(D) The discontinuation of clonidine
(E) A silent myocardial infarction resulting in hemodynamic instability

6. An elderly hypertensive patient on drug treatment develops an anemia, but no source of blood loss can be identified. The evaluation of this patient reveals a positive direct Coombs' test. Which of the following drugs is the most likely cause of this syndrome?

(A) Clonidine
(B) Propranolol
(C) Methyldopa
(D) Prazosin
(E) Reserpine

7. A postmenopausal woman presents with an advanced breast carcinoma that is estrogen receptor–positive. The drug of choice for this patient is

(A) bleomycin
(B) vinblastine
(C) mitomycin
(D) dacarbazine
(E) tamoxifen

8. An 87-year-old man being treated for peripheral vascular disease requires drug therapy for hypertension. All of the following drugs would be acceptable for treating hypertension in this patient EXCEPT

(A) captopril
(B) nifedipine
(C) clonidine
(D) propranolol
(E) hydrochlorothiazide

9. Many elderly persons require treatment for chronic simple (wide-angle) glaucoma. All of the following drugs are used to treat this type of glaucoma EXCEPT

(A) epinephrine
(B) echothiophate
(C) homatropine
(D) timolol
(E) pilocarpine

10. An elderly diabetic patient with an atonic neurogenic bladder is best treated with which of the following medications?

(A) Oxybutynin
(B) Benztropine
(C) Propantheline
(D) Phenylpropanolamine
(E) Bethanechol

11. A 67-year-old man is found to have tachypnea, pitting edema, neck vein distension, and an audible S_3. A chest x-ray shows pulmonary vascular congestion and a large heart. Which of the following diuretic agents is the best medication for this patient?

(A) Mannitol
(B) Hydrochlorothiazide
(C) Bumetanide
(D) Triamterene
(E) Spironolactone

12. Ibuprofen, now available as an over-the-counter analgesic, can cause all of the following adverse effects EXCEPT

(A) impairment of renal function
(B) interference with the drug treatment of hypertension
(C) exacerbation of congestive heart failure symptoms
(D) analgesic nephropathy
(E) acute interstitial nephritis

13. Beta-adrenergic blocking agents cause more serious side effects in elderly patients than in younger patients. All of the following disorders can be worsened in elderly patients treated with β blockers EXCEPT

(A) AV nodal disease
(B) long QT syndrome
(C) peripheral vascular disease
(D) borderline heart failure
(E) reactive airway disease

14. Which of the following characteristics of pharmacologic agents allows them to cross the blood–brain barrier easily?

(A) The ability to bind well to plasma proteins
(B) The ability to ionize readily at physiologic pH
(C) The ability to pass easily through intercellular pores
(D) Lipid solubility
(E) Molecular weight in the intermediate range

15. Aldomet is an antihypertensive agent commonly used in the elderly and an important cause of autoimmune hemolysis. All of the following statements concerning aldomet and autoimmune hemolysis are true EXCEPT

(A) a significant number (as high as 20%) of patients taking aldomet develop a positive direct Coombs' test
(B) clinical hemolysis is infrequent in patients taking aldomet
(C) in patients in whom overt hemolysis is caused by aldomet, the Coombs' test remains positive for several months following discontinuation of the drug
(D) hemolysis occurs by the immune complex mechanism
(E) extravascular hemolysis is more common than intravascular hemolysis

16. All of the following cardiovascular effects are caused by therapeutic dosages of tricyclic antidepressants EXCEPT

(A) conduction delays
(B) orthostatic hypotension
(C) increased ventricular irritability
(D) decreased myocardial contractility
(E) bradycardia

17. Which of the following classes of drugs has the most significant effect on short- and long-term memory in the elderly?

(A) Phenothiazines
(B) Tricyclic antidepressants
(C) Benzodiazepines
(D) MAO inhibitors
(E) Butyrophenones

18. A commonly prescribed drug that may cause parkinsonism is

(A) dipyridamole
(B) imipramine
(C) ranitidine
(D) metoclopramide
(E) clofibrate

19. A hypertensive crisis may be seen in an elderly patient who is taking a drug from which of the following classes?

(A) Tricyclic antidepressants
(B) Barbiturates
(C) Narcotic analgesics
(D) MAO inhibitors
(E) Phenothiazines

Directions: The groups of questions below consist of an introductory premise or case data followed by four statements that pertain to the information given. Indicate whether each statement is **true** or **false**.

Questions 20–23

A 68-year-old smoker who is taking cimetidine for ulcer symptoms requires treatment for COPD. The management of COPD in this patient could be complicated by the following drug interactions.

20. The inhibition of terbutaline metabolism by nicotine

21. The inhibition of theophylline metabolism by cimetidine

22. The enhancement of theophylline metabolism by nicotine

23. The enhancement of theophylline metabolism by terbutaline

Questions 24–27

The following statements describe antidepressant therapy in the elderly.

24. Treatment should be initiated at a very low dosage because of exaggerated sensitivity to side effects

25. Amitriptyline rarely produces sedation, even at moderately high dosages

26. Interactions of MAO inhibitors with foods or other drugs can be especially serious

27. Trazodone predictably produces dry mouth, even at low dosages

Questions 28–31

A 72-year-old woman is seen for a repeat fasting plasma glucose level, which is found to be 305 mg/dl. In the past year, this patient has had plasma glucose levels of 240–280 mg/dl and has been encouraged to watch her diet for excessive caloric intake. Today, as during other office visits, she has no complaints of polyuria or polydipsia. The following therapeutic approaches would be reasonable at this time.

28. A regimen of split-dose (A.M. and P.M.) NPH insulin

29. A prescription for chlorpropamide at a low, once daily dosage

30. A prescription for an 1800-calorie ADA diet

31. A prescription for glipizide at a low, once daily dosage

Questions 32–35

Parkinson's disease affects as many as 1% of people over 70 years of age. The following statements describe the treatment of this disorder.

32. Anticholinergic agents (e.g., benztropine) are effective treatment because they counter unopposed cholinergic activity in dopamine-depleted neurons

33. Combination treatment with levodopa and carbidopa (Sinemet) is effective because carbidopa increases permeability of the blood–brain barrier to levodopa

34. "Drug holiday" (i.e., temporary withdrawal of Sinemet) is the appropriate treatment for levodopa-related complications

35. Amantadine, an antiviral agent also effective in Parkinson's disease, interferes with the action of levodopa; thus, the two agents should not be used in combination

Questions 36–39

Warfarin is an oral anticoagulant commonly used in the elderly for treatment of thrombotic events. Chronic anticoagulant therapy in these patients often is complicated by interaction with other drugs they may be taking. An increased hypoprothrombinemic effect of warfarin is caused by concomitant use of the following drugs.

36. Cimetidine

37. Aspirin

38. Furosemide

39. Pentobarbital

Questions 40–43

Benzodiazepines are useful drugs in the elderly due to their effectiveness as hypnotics, antianxiety agents, and anticonvulsants. The following benzodiazepines are preferred for elderly patients because they do not produce active metabolites.

40. Lorazepam

41. Flurazepam

42. Diazepam

43. Triazolam

Questions 44–47

The following drugs affect the renal clearance of uric acid.

44. Allopurinol

45. Sulfinpyrazone

46. Colchicine

47. Aspirin

ANSWERS AND EXPLANATIONS

1. The answer is E. Significant changes in body composition occur with advancing age. In general, elderly people are smaller than younger adults, owing to a gradual but significant decrease in muscle mass combined with a decline in total body water. This considerable decrease in lean body mass is offset somewhat by a significant increase in body fat. These body composition changes can cause major alterations in drug distribution in the elderly patient. The decreased muscle mass can lead to too-high drug dosages, the decreased body water can lead to increased and possibly toxic effects with water-soluble drugs, and the increased body fat can lead to decreased but prolonged effects with fat-soluble drugs. Although hepatic metabolism of drugs is clinically difficult to predict, most aspects of liver function decline with aging. Reasons for this include decreased liver weight and volume, reduced splanchnic blood flow, and decreased microsomal enzyme activity within hepatocytes. Advancing age also is associated with several anatomic and physiologic changes in the kidney, which lead to decreased drug clearance. One cause of reduced glomerular filtration is decreased renal blood flow secondary to an age-related decline in cardiac output.

2. The answer is D. Bethanechol is a cholinergic agonist; activation of the cholinergic nerves increases LES tone. In adequate amounts (25 mg 3 times daily), bethanechol increases LES pressure, thus preventing regurgitation. Metoclopramide is another drug that increases LES pressure. Substances known to decrease LES pressure are alcohol, anticholinergic agents, antihistamines, nitrates, methylxanthines, morphine, nicotine, and some foods (e.g., chocolate).

3. The answer is A. Ipratropium, an atropine-like bronchodilator, is a quaternary ammonium compound with low lipid solubility. It is particularly effective in the treatment of chronic bronchitis; however, in an elderly man with benign prostatic hyperplasia, this anticholinergic agent may aggravate urinary retention. Buspirone and glyburide have no action on the genitourinary tract. Timolol blocks β-adrenergic receptors in the bladder and could allow α-adrenergic dominance; however, this is seen primarily with oral administration. Hydroxyzine has anticholinergic activity, but urinary retention rarely is reported.

4. The answer is B. Although β-adrenergic blocking agents (e.g., propranolol, metoprolol, nadolol) are useful in the management of hypertension and the prophylaxis of angina, these drugs are potentially hazardous in patients with congestive heart failure because they decrease heart rate and cardiac output. Calcium-channel blocking agents (e.g., nifedipine, verapamil) are effective therapy for angina because of their vasodilating effect on coronary arteries. Verapamil, although having similar pharmacologic activity to nifedipine, is relatively contraindicated in patients with heart failure, because it has negative inotropic and chronotropic activity and slows AV conduction. In addition to dilating the coronary arteries, nifedipine may reduce afterload and peripheral blood pressure, which mitigates its negative inotropic effects.

5. The answer is A. Although a silent myocardial infarction cannot be ruled out entirely in this patient, based on the data presented it is somewhat unlikely in the absence of prior coronary artery disease or a history of anginal symptoms. The onset of fatigue and shortness of breath suggests that the patient has congestive heart failure. Certainly, the doubling of the propranolol dosage in this patient could precipitate these heart failure symptoms via negative inotropic and chronotropic effects. Even without causing heart failure, propranolol is known for its ability to cause fatigue in some patients.

6. The answer is C. Clonidine, propranolol, methyldopa, prazosin, and reserpine all are appropriate drugs for the treatment of hypertension in adult patients. A possible risk associated with the use of methyldopa, however, is the development of a positive direct Coombs' test, with a smaller risk being a drug-induced hemolytic anemia.

7. The answer is E. The growth of certain breast carcinomas depends on the presence of estrogens, and, in such cases, appropriate therapy can greatly reduce tumor cell proliferation. Antiestrogenic agents, such as tamoxifen, compete with estrogen for the cytoplasmic estrogen receptor and, thus, block the growth of estrogen-dependent tumors. Bleomycin, mitomycin, and vinblastine are natural products that have little activity against breast carcinomas. Dacarbazine (DTIC) is a triazene alkylating agent that is effective against melanomas but is not effective against breast carcinomas.

8. The answer is D. In peripheral vascular disease, blood circulation can be compromised further with β-adrenergic blocking drugs such as propranolol; β-receptor blockade allows α-receptor–mediated vasoconstriction to dominate. Captopril, an ACE inhibitor, and nifedipine, a calcium-channel blocker, are gaining acceptance as antihypertensive agents in the elderly. Clonidine and hydrochlorothiazide have been used for many years to treat hypertension in the aged patient.

9. The answer is C. Glaucoma refers to a group of eye diseases characterized by an increase in intraocular pressure, which results in damage to the optic disk and vision defects. Primary glaucoma is divided into two types: chronic simple (wide-angle) glaucoma, which is by far the most common in the elderly, and acute congestive (narrow-angle) glaucoma. A variety of drugs are available for reducing intraocular pressure in wide-angle glaucoma. Epinephrine, a sympathomimetic agent, relaxes the ciliary muscle and dilates the pupil; echothiophate, an anticholinesterase agent, lowers resistance to the outflow of aqueous humor; timolol, a β-adrenergic blocking agent, decreases aqueous humor formation; and pilocarpine, a parasympathomimetic agent, produces miosis and chronic reduction in intraocular pressure. Homatropine, an anticholinergic agent, is not used in the treatment of wide-angle glaucoma and is contraindicated in narrow-angle glaucoma, because it dilates the pupil and would increase intraocular pressure by obstructing outflow of aqueous humor.

10. The answer is E. Elderly diabetic patients often develop neurogenic bladder as a neuropathic complication. These patients cannot sense bladder fullness and have overflow incontinence. The primary treatment is to teach the patient to void routinely. In advanced disease, cholinergic drugs (e.g., bethanechol 25–50 mg 3 or 4 times daily) are given to stimulate contraction of the smooth muscle of the bladder. Oxybutynin, benztropine, and propantheline are anticholinergic and antispasmodic drugs used to control involuntary contractions of the bladder. Phenylpropanolamine, an α-adrenergic receptor stimulant, increases internal urethral sphincter tone and is used to manage stress incontinence. All of these drugs should be used with caution in the elderly. Bethanechol can cause hypotension; anticholinergic agents can cause tachycardia and hypertension and can precipitate glaucoma.

11. The answer is C. This patient has clinical evidence of pulmonary edema—severe congestive heart failure. Without prompt and effective treatment, the impaired oxygenation in this patient can lead to death. The goal of therapy is to improve oxygenation, to reduce left ventricular filling pressure, and to increase forward cardiac output. A potent, rapid-acting loop diuretic (e.g., bumetanide, furosemide), given intravenously, causes immediate venodilation and, thus, a decrease in preload; it also promotes prompt diuresis in most cases. The moderately potent thiazide diuretics (e.g., hydrochlorothiazide, chlorthalidone) would not provide the immediate diuretic response that is needed. Even less potent are the potassium-sparing diuretics (e.g., spironolactone, triamterene), which are appropriate for treatment of congestive heart failure only when used in conjunction with a loop or thiazide diuretic. Mannitol is an osmotic diuretic that is contraindicated in patients with severe cardiac decompensation, because it causes acute expansion of the extracellular fluid volume.

12. The answer is D. Ibuprofen is a widely used nonsteroidal anti-inflammatory drug (NSAID) that is regarded as equivalent to aspirin in analgesic as well as anti-inflammatory properties. However, it can cause reversible impairment of renal function (just like other NSAIDs) due to its effects on renal prostaglandin synthesis, especially in patients whose renal blood flow is dependent on prostaglandin synthesis because of reduced effective arterial blood volume. The most common diseases associated with reduced effective arterial perfusion are nephrosis, cirrhosis, and congestive heart failure. In addition, elderly patients are much more likely to suffer reversible impairment of renal function from NSAIDs. These agents also can cause sodium and water retention, thus interfering with the treatment of hypertension and congestive heart failure and, possibly, causing peripheral edema. Although ibuprofen is one of the agents that occasionally can cause acute interstitial nephritis (a condition characterized by fever, eosinophiluria, proteinuria, and renal interstitial inflammatory infiltrates), it has not yet been shown to cause analgesic nephropathy. Phenacetin is the only drug clearly associated with this disease, usually in combination with other analgesic agents.

13. The answer is B. The β-adrenergic blocking agents are highly effective drugs for managing certain cardiovascular disorders; recent studies have shown β blockers to reduce both the incidence of reinfarction and the number of deaths due to myocardial infarction. These drugs are not without significant side effects, however, which may be particularly serious in the elderly. In particular, β blockers may exacerbate such existing disorders as AV nodal disease, borderline pump failure, peripheral vascular disease, and reactive airway disease—all of which may not be clinically evident in elderly persons. Long QT syndrome is an abnormal prolongation of the QT interval, which is associated with syncope and sudden death due to cardiac arrhythmias. The prolonged QT interval can be an inherited disorder or can be acquired as a result of drugs, electrolyte imbalances, or CNS lesions. This syndrome can be seen in the elderly and in many cases is treated successfully with propranolol (a β blocker).

14. The answer is D. The blood–brain barrier protects the brain from foreign substances. Agents that are lipid soluble, that are not ionized at physiologic pH, and that bind poorly to plasma proteins are better able to diffuse across this barrier. The physiologic basis for the blood–brain barrier appears to be the tight junctions between the endothelial cells that line the capillaries of the brain. There are no intercellular pores or pinocytotic vesicles in these capillaries for drugs to pass through. In general, agents of lower molecular weight cross the blood–brain barrier more easily than ones of intermediate or high molecular weight.

15. The answer is D. Aldomet, like levodopa, can induce hemolysis but not by the immune complex mechanism. In aldomet-related hemolysis, an antibody is directed against erythrocyte Rh components, and erythrocytes coated with this IgG or IgM antibody are removed in the spleen and reticuloendothelial system. Aldomet probably functions by inhibiting suppressor T cells, allowing B cells to produce autoantibodies. About 20% of patients, therefore, do develop a positive direct Coombs' test (i.e., evidence of erythrocytes coated with IgG), although only about 1% develop clinical hemolysis. The Coombs' positivity is slow to resolve upon discontinuation of aldomet, because impaired suppressor T cell function is slow to return to normal.

16. The answer is E. Tricyclic antidepressants produce a number of effects on the cardiovascular system. The most widely known effect is on conduction, since these drugs may cause progression of a preexisting conduction defect due to their quinidine-like effect. The anticholinergic reactions caused by tricyclic agents include tachycardia (not bradycardia), which can be a particular problem for older people with angina or congestive heart failure. Also, there is evidence that these drugs have a negative inotropic effect on the heart. Orthostatic hypotension is believed to be related to the α-adrenergic blocking activity of tricyclics. Ventricular arrhythmias also can occur, particularly when bundle branch block is present or when an overdose of the drugs is taken.

17. The answer is C. Although low-potency phenothiazines and some antidepressants may produce sedation, they have not yet been demonstrated to have significant effects on memory. Benzodiazepines often are used to calm agitated demented patients, particularly in the hospital or nursing home setting; however, their use is not without some risk. Short- and long-term memory is more significantly affected by benzodiazepines (e.g., lorazepam) than by drugs from any of the other classifications listed. In addition, the sedation produced by benzodiazepines decreases attention, thus making cognitively impaired persons even less likely to pick up important environmental cues.

18. The answer is D. The drugs that cause parkinsonism either block the dopamine$_2$ (D_2) receptors or deplete the dopamine stores. Antipsychotic drugs (e.g., chlorpromazine, haloperidol) and metoclopramide (a drug used in the treatment of upper gastrointestinal motility disorders) are examples of D_2-receptor blocking drugs; reserpine is an example of a dopamine-depleting drug. Dipyridamole, imipramine, ranitidine, and clofibrate do not cause extrapyramidal disorders.

19. The answer is D. MAO inhibitors can interact with sympathomimetic amines, especially indirect acting ones (e.g., amphetamine, tyramine), and with certain foods that contain high amounts of tyramine (e.g., cheese, beer). As a result, catecholamines are released from nerve terminals, producing the hypertensive crisis. Tricyclic antidepressants, barbiturates, narcotic analgesics, and phenothiazines can cause hypotension, not hypertension.

20–23. The answers are: 20-F, 21-T, 22-T, 23-F. Bronchodilation is the most effective therapy for COPD. Two major classes of bronchodilators currently available are methylxanthines (e.g., theophylline) and β-adrenergic agonists (e.g., terbutaline); these agents may be used separately or in combination. Theophylline metabolism is subject to several factors that affect the dosage requirements in geriatric patients. Nicotine accelerates the hepatic metabolism of theophylline; therefore, dosage requirements for smoking patients would be expected to be higher than those for nonsmoking patients. In contrast, cimetidine slows the metabolism of theophylline and leads to higher than expected plasma levels. Terbutaline is not known to interact with nicotine or theophylline.

24–27. The answers are: 24-T, 25-F, 26-T, 27-F. Side effects of antidepressant therapy are exaggerated in elderly patients, and, therefore, treatment usually is started at lower dosages than those used in younger patients. Sedation is a common problem for patients of all ages who are treated with antidepressants; this would be especially true in geriatric patients on moderately high dosages of amitryptyline. Hypertensive crisis can be seen when patients on MAO inhibitors eat tyramine-containing foods or use sympathomimetic drugs. This side effect would be especially serious in an elderly person with cardiovascular or cerebrovascular disease. Undesirable anticholinergic effects of tricyclic agents, such as dry mouth, occur less frequently in patients receiving trazodone, a newly available triazolopyridine derivative.

28–31. The answers are: 28-F, 29-F, 30-T, 31-T. Split-dose, intermediate-acting insulin treatment is more appropriate for younger diabetic patients who are poorly controlled on once daily insulin injections. This regimen poses too high a risk of hypoglycemia in an elderly person such as the one described here.

Chlorpropamide is a long-acting oral hypoglycemic agent that should not be used in the elderly, because drug accumulation can lead to sustained hypoglycemia. Also, fluid retention can result in hyponatremia and congestive heart failure.

Probably the best therapeutic approach to this patient at this time is to attempt careful dietary control with an 1800-calorie ADA diet. This regimen may be effective alone and does not carry risks of side effects.

An oral hypoglycemic agent might be appropriate at this stage if the patient were unable to comply with stricter dietary regulation. Glipizide, a second-generation sulfonylurea drug, has fewer side effects and fewer drug interactions in the elderly than a first-generation drug such as chlorpropamide.

32–35. The answers are: 32-T, 33-F, 34-F, 35-F. Anticholinergic agents partially restore the balance between dopaminergic and cholinergic effects in the CNS of patients with Parkinson's disease, leading to improved motor function. Before the advent of levodopa therapy, anticholinergic drugs were the primary treatment for Parkinson's disease.

Carbidopa does not affect permeability of the blood–brain barrier; rather, it prevents the peripheral conversion of levodopa to dopamine, which cannot cross the blood–brain barrier. Thus, using carbidopa with levodopa allows for lower dosages of levodopa and reduces levodopa side effects.

"Drug holidays" are associated with thrombophlebitis, severe rigidity, and aspiration pneumonia as consequences of the lost effect of levodopa. Although some patients benefit temporarily from the apparent return of dopamine receptor sensitivity provided by such holidays, sustained benefit is too infrequent to justify the consequences in most patients.

Amantadine increases dopamine release from remaining substantia nigra neurons. Its effects do not antagonize those of levodopa; rather, the effects of the two drugs are additive.

36–39. The answers are: 36-T, 37-T, 38-T, 39-F. The chronic use of warfarin always should be approached with a complete understanding of potential drug interactions. Among the clinically significant interactions with warfarin are those that primarily affect its metabolism or its protein binding. Drugs that inhibit warfarin metabolism (e.g., cimetidine, disulfiram) increase the amount of drug in plasma available for pharmacologic activity and, therefore, increase its hypoprothrombinemic effect. Drugs that are significantly bound to plasma albumin (e.g., furosemide, ethacrynic acid) may compete with warfarin or displace it from sites on the protein, producing more free drug and, thus, an enhanced pharmacologic response. Concomitant use of aspirin can have severe hemorrhagic consequences due to the combined effects of decreased fibrin formation (with warfarin) and decreased platelet aggregation (with aspirin). In addition, the hypoprothrombinemic response to warfarin is increased in patients who take large amounts of aspirin every day. Like all barbiturates, pentobarbital enhances warfarin metabolism, thus decreasing the amount of drug available for pharmacologic activity.

40–43. The answers are: 40-T, 41-F, 42-F, 43-T. When treating elderly patients for anxiety or insomnia, benzodiazepines that do not produce long-acting metabolites are chosen over ones that do. Flurazepam and diazepam have active metabolites that prolong their effects; accumulation of the active by-products can cause excessive sedation and incoordination, with a greater potential for accidents. The short-acting benzodiazepines (e.g., lorazepam, oxazepam, triazolam) are preferred, as they do not appear to have active metabolites and, thus, have transient effects. The elderly are extremely sensitive to hypnotics and should be given them only for a short period of time and for specific indications. All of these agents should be used carefully in geriatric patients because of paradoxical excitability or sleeplessness.

44–47. The answers are: 44-F, 45-T, 46-F, 47-T. Allopurinol does not affect the renal clearance of uric acid, but it does interfere with uric acid synthesis by inhibiting xanthine oxidase, the enzyme that converts xanthine and hypoxanthine to uric acid. Sulfinpyrazone and probenecid are widely used uricosuric agents that work by blocking renal tubular reabsorption of urate. Colchicine has an anti-inflammatory effect in gout, but it does not affect uric acid synthesis or clearance. Salicylates (e.g., aspirin) are anti-inflammatory agents that do affect the renal clearance of urate, albeit unpredictably; at low doses salicylates enhance urate reabsorption, but at higher doses they block urate reuptake by the renal tubules. Acute gouty attacks can be prolonged by fluctuations in urate levels, so salicylates typically are not used to treat acute gout. Sustained, high-dose salicylate therapy occasionally is employed to prevent acute attacks (anti-inflammatory effect) and to lower serum urate levels (uricosuric effect) in patients with chronic gout.

2 Gastrointestinal Disorders

QUESTIONS

Directions: Each question below contains five suggested answers. Choose the **one best** response to each question.

1. Elderly patients frequently complain of disorders involving the gastrointestinal tract. All of the following statements characterize these complaints EXCEPT

(A) most gastrointestinal complaints by elderly patients are the result of emotional or functional factors
(B) when functional factors are the cause of complaints, they relate to gastric motility or secretion
(C) an organic cause generally is found upon investigation of constipation
(D) a preoccupation with foods and elimination is common among elderly patients
(E) recurrence of symptoms often is related to emotional stress

2. A 55-year-old man who travels extensively for work is seen because he has been vomiting bright-red blood. He has experienced no other symptoms, however. The only medication he uses is acetaminophen for headache, and he rarely drinks alcohol. In the hospital, this patient loses an estimated 5 units of blood prior to endoscopy. The most likely diagnosis is

(A) gastritis
(B) duodenal ulcer
(C) esophagitis
(D) Mallory-Weiss tear
(E) esophageal varices

3. An elderly man is brought to the emergency room because of sudden massive bleeding from the rectum. The bleeding is most likely due to

(A) colonic carcinoma
(B) diverticulosis
(C) diverticulitis
(D) ulcerative colitis
(E) colonic polyps

4. Constipation is a common complaint of elderly persons. All of the following factors contribute to this problem EXCEPT

(A) increased gastrointestinal transit time
(B) laxative abuse
(C) ignoring the urge to defecate
(D) poor dietary habits
(E) sedentary lifestyle

5. An elderly woman is admitted to the hospital with weakness, anemia, weight loss, and a palpable abdominal mass. Barium enema and colonoscopy confirm the diagnosis of a malignancy. The most likely anatomic site of the cancer is the

(A) rectum
(B) sigmoid colon
(C) left colon
(D) transverse colon
(E) cecum

6. All of the following statements describe the diagnosis and treatment of acute pancreatitis in the elderly EXCEPT

(A) serum amylase levels are elevated during an acute attack
(B) renal clearance of amylase is elevated during an acute attack
(C) ultrasonography is used to exclude gallstones as a cause of the acute attack
(D) therapy includes nasogastric suction to drain gastric secretions
(E) morphine is given to relieve the severe pain that accompanies an acute attack

7. In a 70-year-old patient with a 2-week history of jaundice and no abdominal pain, a markedly distended gallbladder seen on ultrasonography is most likely secondary to which of the following diagnoses?

(A) Choledocholithiasis
(B) Chronic pancreatitis
(C) Pancreatic carcinoma
(D) Acute cholecystitis
(E) Alcoholic hepatitis

8. Cancer of the esophagus is primarily a disease of elderly men. All of the following statements characterize esophageal cancer EXCEPT

(A) esophageal cancer usually is of the squamous-cell type
(B) esophageal cancer usually occurs in association with benign strictures
(C) alcoholism frequently is associated with esophageal cancer
(D) dysphagia for liquids, cough, and hoarseness are early manifestations of esophageal cancer
(E) a steady, boring pain signals mediastinal involvement and an inoperable lesion

9. Pancreatitis in a nonalcoholic elderly patient is most likely due to

(A) pancreatic carcinoma
(B) gallstones
(C) hydrochlorothiazide therapy
(D) duodenal ulcer
(E) hypertriglyceridemia

10. The lower esophagus of a patient is inadvertently perforated during esophagoscopy. A barium swallow done immediately after perforation demonstrates that a small amount of barium is leaking into the left pleural space. What is the most acceptable method of treatment?

(A) Observation plus antibiotics
(B) Insertion of a left chest tube
(C) Insertion of a left chest tube plus antibiotics
(D) Prolonged esophageal intubation
(E) Drainage and surgical repair of the injury

11. All of the following statements concerning hiatal hernia in the elderly are true EXCEPT

(A) more often than not, hiatal hernia is present in persons over age 70
(B) the presence of a hiatal hernia does not affect LES function
(C) the presence of a hiatal hernia delays gastric emptying and promotes reflux
(D) penetrating esophageal ulcers are a common complication of hiatal hernia
(E) surgical management should be considered in resistant cases

12. A 72-year-old man is admitted to the hospital with massive, bright-red rectal bleeding. He recently had a barium enema that demonstrated no diverticular or space-occupying lesion. Nasogastric suction reveals no blood but does produce yellow bile. The patient continues to bleed. What is the most useful diagnostic procedure at this point?

(A) Repeat barium enema
(B) Colonoscopy
(C) Upper gastrointestinal series
(D) Mesenteric angiography
(E) Enteroclysis

13. Pancreatic inflammation is common among elderly alcoholics. Which of the following is a late clinical feature of acute pancreatitis?

(A) Diminished or absent bowel sounds
(B) Epigastric fullness or mass
(C) Fever
(D) Nausea and vomiting
(E) Back pain

14. A 68-year-old chronic alcoholic with known cirrhosis is noted to have a mass in the right lobe of his liver and an elevated α-fetoprotein level. What is the most likely diagnosis?

(A) Hepatocellular adenoma
(B) Hepatocellular carcinoma
(C) Metastatic carcinoma of the colon
(D) Hepatic abscess
(E) Focal nodular hyperplasia

15. Appendicitis often has an atypical presentation in elderly patients, which leads to a delayed diagnosis with an increased risk of perforation. An elderly patient with appendicitis is likely to have all of the following signs and symptoms EXCEPT

(A) rebound tenderness and guarding
(B) abdominal distension
(C) nausea and anorexia
(D) constipation
(E) low-grade fever

16. A 60-year-old, otherwise healthy man is hospitalized for massive bleeding from the lower gastrointestinal tract. His blood pressure is stabilized with intravenous fluids, but the patient continues to have frequent stools containing bright-red blood. The best initial treatment of this patient is

(A) emergency laparotomy and total colectomy with ileoproctostomy
(B) emergency laparotomy and colostomy with operative endoscopy
(C) arteriography to identify the bleeding site after anoscopy and sigmoidoscopy have ruled out a distal site
(D) infusion of vitamin K and fresh frozen plasma
(E) colonic irrigation with iced saline solution

17. Peptic ulcer disease is common in the geriatric population. All of the following statements characterize this disease as it occurs in the elderly EXCEPT

(A) elderly persons who smoke are at an increased risk for peptic ulcers
(B) giant ulcers occur more commonly in the duodenum than in the stomach
(C) weight loss and anorexia may be the only symptoms
(D) perforation often occurs in patients with no prior history of peptic ulcer symptoms
(E) perforation may occur in the absence of abdominal pain and rigidity

Questions 18 and 19

A 70-year-old man presents with severe left lower quadrant pain, a temperature of 102° F, and a history of pain on defecation. Initial examination of this patient reveals a blood pressure of 105/70 mm Hg, a pulse of 112/min, and mildly labored breathing. Abdominal examination reveals diminished bowel sounds and left lower quadrant tenderness without rebound.

18. All of the following are appropriate measures to be taken at this time EXCEPT

(A) administration of clindamycin and gentamicin
(B) administration of cefoxitin
(C) strict bowel rest
(D) flexible sigmoidoscopy
(E) barium enema

19. On rectal examination, the patient is noted to have tenderness to the left of the prostate gland. Urinalysis reveals 10–15 white blood cells per high-power field but no bacteria or blood. Based on these findings, what is the most accurate conclusion?

(A) The diagnosis is prostatitis
(B) The diagnosis is diverticulosis
(C) The diagnosis is renal tuberculosis
(D) The diagnosis is intra-abdominal abscess
(E) Urine culture is necessary to distinguish between these possibilities

Directions: The groups of questions below consist of an introductory premise or case data followed by four statements that pertain to the information given. Indicate whether each statement is **true** or **false**.

Questions 20–23

Ischemic colitis is due to inadequate arterial blood supply to the colon. The following statements describe the pathophysiology, clinical manifestations, and diagnosis of ischemic colitis.

20. The rectum and sigmoid colon usually are spared due to their generous blood supply

21. The most commonly affected site is the hepatic flexure

22. The symptoms include bloody diarrhea and abdominal pain and distension

23. The diagnosis is suggested by thumb-printing on barium enema

Questions 24–27

Peptic ulcer disease is on the rise in the elderly population. Although duodenal ulcers are more common than gastric ulcers, the latter carry the risk of being malignant and are the cause of more deaths. Radiography is a useful tool for screening gastric ulcers. The following signs are radiographic criteria for benign gastric ulcers.

24. Ulcer crater extending beyond the gastric wall

25. Gastric folds radiating into the ulcer crater

26. Collar of edema surrounding the ulcer base

27. Stiff, nonpliable gastric wall near the ulcer crater

Questions 28–31

An elderly patient suddenly experiences painless massive hematochezia. The following statements describe this problem.

28. Diverticulosis is a much more common cause of this syndrome than colonic angiodysplasia

29. Barium enema likely will establish the cause of bleeding

30. Sigmoidoscopy is the most appropriate initial diagnostic procedure if the bleeding stops

31. Most patients who bleed once from diverticulosis will experience another bleeding episode in the future

Questions 32–35

Adenomatous polyps of the colon are premalignant lesions. The following statements describe factors that determine risk for adenocarcinoma in these lesions.

32. Polyps located in the right colon are more likely to be malignant

33. Polyps smaller than 1 cm are unlikely to be malignant

34. Villous adenomas rarely are malignant

35. Sessile polyps are more likely to be malignant than pedunculated ones

Questions 36–39

Bleeding is a common complication of peptic ulcer disease. The following statements accurately describe this potentially life-threatening problem.

36. The first priority in treating patients with bleeding ulcers is to locate the site of bleeding

37. Most patients with bleeding ulcers respond to medical treatment alone

38. The mortality rate is higher in gastric than in duodenal ulcer disease

39. The mortality rate does not rise with increasing age

Questions 40–43

Atrophic gastritis is classified as type A or type B, the latter being the more common form. The following features characterize type B atrophic gastritis.

40. Marked atrophy and inflammation of the antral mucosa

41. Association with autoimmune diseases

42. Deficiency of intrinsic factor, which can lead to pernicious anemia

43. Chronic blood loss

Questions 44–47

The incidence of colonic diverticula increases with age. The following age-related changes in the colon are believed to contribute to the pathogenesis of diverticular disease.

44. Altered chemical structure of collagen fibers in the muscularis

45. Increased compliance of the colonic wall

46. Increased pressure gradient across the colonic lumen

47. Disturbed colonic motility due to neuron degeneration

Questions 48–51

Acute cholecystitis occurs with greater frequency in older persons and carries a higher risk of complications, including death. The following are reasons for increased morbidity and mortality in an elderly patient.

48. A delay in the diagnosis due to an atypical presentation

49. The use of ultrasonography for the diagnosis, which is less reliable in the acute setting than oral cholecystography

50. A delay of longer than 2 months in performing cholecystectomy after an episode of acute cholecystitis

51. Failure to use choledochotomy in conjunction with cholecystectomy

ANSWERS AND EXPLANATIONS

1. The answer is C. Gastrointestinal disorders account for a large number of complaints in the elderly population. Most of these complaints are of a functional nature, without any demonstrable organic basis. Typically, the complaints relate to poor eating habits, inadequate bowel habits, and a preoccupation with foods and elimination. A fear of death and disease and an apprehension of colon cancer also are factors to be considered in dealing with elderly patients who complain of gastrointestinal disorders.

2. The answer is B. Massive upper gastrointestinal hemorrhage usually is due to a bleeding source proximal to the ligament of Treitz. Determining the anatomic site of bleeding is aided considerably by a careful medical history and a detailed chronicle of the patient's symptoms. The most common cause of bleeding is peptic ulcer disease, and this bleeding may be massive if due to a posterior duodenal ulcer that erodes into the gastroduodenal artery. Hemorrhage often is the first manifestation of a peptic ulcer. Erosive gastritis may cause bleeding, but usually it is in the clinical setting of chronic aspirin use or alcohol ingestion. Esophagitis is another possible source of upper gastrointestinal bleeding, but it causes chronic blood loss, not abrupt massive bleeding. A Mallory-Weiss tear usually presents initially as retching, then nonbloody vomiting, followed by hematemesis. Esophageal varices may cause abrupt bleeding in patients with associated portal hypertension (usually due to alcoholic cirrhosis).

3. The answer is B. Diverticulosis is one of the most common causes of massive hemorrhage in the lower gastrointestinal tract; another common cause is angiodysplasia (i.e., arteriovenous malformation) of the right colon. Bleeding due to diverticulosis typically begins without warning, is brisk and profuse, and ceases spontaneously. In contrast, bleeding that is associated with colonic carcinoma or polyps is mild and persistent. Ulcerative colitis often is associated with bloody diarrhea but not with massive rectal bleeding. Diverticulitis also is not associated with massive bleeding.

4. The answer is A. Although many elderly persons complain of constipation, this problem is not necessarily a result of advancing age. Studies have shown that the gastrointestinal transit time in older persons is not significantly different from that in younger persons. Other factors, however, do contribute to constipation in elderly persons, such as poor eating habits (especially inadequate intake of water and fiber-rich foods), decreased physical activity, and repeatedly ignoring the urge to defecate, which leads to a decreased awareness of a full rectum. Abuse of laxatives, particularly stimulant laxatives (e.g., phenolphthalein, bisacodyl), can lead to a damaged colon and consequent constipation. Elderly persons are frequent abusers of laxatives.

5. The answer is E. Colorectal cancer is an increasing problem in developed countries, where diets typically are high in red meat and low in fiber. The incidence of these cancers increases with age and is highest in persons who are 70–80 years old. The clinical presentation of colorectal cancers varies with the location and size of the tumor. Tumors in the right colon, including the cecum, are likely to be silent until they become very large. They cause heme-positive stools from a slow, chronic blood loss. The resultant anemia is so insidious in its onset that it often does not cause symptoms until late in the course. Patients present with iron deficiency anemia, fatigue, weight loss, or a palpable abdominal mass. In contrast, tumors in the left colon are more obvious in their presentation, with increasing obstruction causing constipation, rectal bleeding, and abdominal pain. Tumors in the rectum often present as occult blood in the stool, a change in bowel habits, and fecal urgency upon arising.

6. The answer is E. The pancreas is the source of several digestive enzymes, including amylase. During an acute pancreatic attack, serum amylase levels are elevated—the hallmark of pancreatitis. Because other digestive disorders are associated with high serum amylase levels, it is useful to measure the renal clearance of amylase when acute pancreatitis is suspected, as the ratio of amylase clearance to creatinine clearance is markedly elevated in these patients. Ultrasonography may be used to exclude gallstones as a cause of symptoms. Treatment includes gastric measures to rest the pancreas (i.e., nasogastric suction, restriction of oral feeding, or draining gastric secretions) and intravenous administration of fluids and electrolytes. Analgesics should be provided for relief of pain; however, morphine is contraindicated for pain relief because it causes spasm of the sphincter of Oddi.

7. The answer is C. Painless jaundice in the presence of a distended gallbladder is most likely secondary to a carcinoma of the head of the pancreas. In patients with common duct stones, chronic pancreatitis and acute cholecystitis, single or multiple episodes of abdominal pain would be typical. Alcoholic hepatitis usually does not cause a distended gallbladder, and the patient would have an associated history of alcohol abuse.

8. The answer is D. Esophageal cancer occurs mainly in the elderly population, with a greater incidence in men than in women. Cases of adenocarcinoma of the esophagus are rare; most esophageal cancer is of the squamous-cell type. Smoking and alcohol consumption have an additive effect in increasing the risk for development of this cancer. Persistent and progressive dysphagia for solids is an early sign. Dysphagia for liquids, cough, hoarseness, and weight loss are later symptoms of the disease. A steady, boring pain is an ominous sign, indicating mediastinal involvement and an inoperable lesion.

9. The answer is B. Gallstones are the most common and important cause of pancreatitis in the elderly. Other, less common, causes include pancreatic carcinoma with obstruction of the pancreatic duct, duodenal ulcer, hypertriglyceridemia, and treatment with such drugs as thiazides and corticosteroids. Acute pancreatitis is associated with alcoholism much less frequently in elderly patients than in younger patients, in whom alcoholism is the principal cause of acute pancreatitis. In any event, a reversible cause should be sought aggressively to prevent the recurrence of acute pancreatitis.

10. The answer is E. Recognized perforation of the esophagus is most safely treated by thoracotomy and repair of the injury with wide drainage, even in an elderly patient who might be at greater risk for complications of general anesthesia. Failure to carry out these measures may result in a life-threatening infection.

11. The answer is D. Hiatal hernia is a very common occurrence in the elderly population; it is an incidental finding on routine radiographic examination in approximately 70% of patients over the age of 70. The hernia generally does not affect the function of the LES but may delay gastric emptying and promote gastroesophageal reflux. A hiatal hernia has little clinical significance except in rare situations in which it causes extreme reflux as a result of delayed gastric emptying. Patients with persistent gastroesophageal reflux and extreme esophagitis should undergo surgical repair of the hernia. Incarcerated hernias are associated with excruciating pain, dysphagia, anemia, and respiratory symptoms. These hernias often simulate myocardial infarctions.

12. The answer is D. The most likely cause of massive lower gastrointestinal bleeding in the absence of diverticula is an angiodysplastic lesion of the colon, particularly the right colon. An upper gastrointestinal series and small bowel studies (enteroclysis) should be done only after an exhaustive colonic workup has failed to demonstrate the source of bleeding. Colonoscopy in the face of massive bleeding is unreliable and difficult and carries the risk of colonic perforation. In addition, it usually will not demonstrate an angiodysplastic lesion. A repeat barium enema also is unlikely to help. The most helpful study in this patient would be selective mesenteric angiography.

13. The answer is B. Acute pancreatitis is a debilitating disease commonly associated with alcoholism; other conditions that predispose to pancreatitis include gallstones, hypercalcemia, hyperlipoproteinemia, and penetrating peptic ulcer. Acute pancreatitis presents as severe midepigastric pain that within a short time radiates through to the back. After the pain peaks in intensity, patients experience nausea and profuse vomiting; fever also develops in many cases. Respiratory distress may follow, accompanied by cyanosis and left-sided pleurisy. Examination usually reveals diminished or absent bowel sounds and pain and bluish discoloration in the periumbilical region due to retroperitoneal bleeding. Late in the attack, an epigastric mass may be palpated, which indicates the presence of a pseudocyst or pancreatic abscess. Pseudocysts are common complications of recurrent pancreatitis in alcoholic patients, abscesses are much less common.

14. The answer is B. The relationship between cirrhosis and primary liver carcinoma is well documented. In adults, the majority of primary liver carcinomas are hepatocellular. A highly sensitive diagnostic indicator of hepatocellular carcinoma is an elevated α-fetoprotein level. This protein is an oncofetal antigen found in the serum of up to 85% of patients with hepatocellular carcinoma. Hepatocellular adenoma and focal nodular hyperplasia are benign tumors that usually occur in women of childbearing age; serum α-fetoprotein levels are normal in these patients. Metastatic disease is much more common than primary hepatic malignancy and in most cases spreads from colorectal cancers; an elevated serum alkaline phosphatase level often is the only hepatic enzyme abnormality in these patients. Hepatic abscess typically is associated with fever, abdominal pain, and sepsis; α-fetoprotein elevations are not characteristic.

15. The answer is A. Appendicitis is not as common in the elderly as in the young, but it has more serious implications in the older age-group. A delay in seeking medical attention and a delayed or incorrect diagnosis due to atypical presentations increase the risk of perforation in older patients and result in a relatively high mortality rate. Elderly patients typically present with vague abdominal discomfort with distension, constipation, nausea, and anorexia. Rebound tenderness and abdominal guarding, which are very common in younger patients, are absent in most elderly patients. In addition, temperatures usually do not exceed 102° F, and leukocyte count often is normal.

16. The answer is C. Arteriography is most often used as the initial step in the evaluation for continued bleeding after anorectal bleeding sources have been eliminated by endoscopy. Arteriography allows identification of diverticular bleeding as well as an angiodysplastic lesion of the right colon. Barium enema also may be used in the initial management, since bleeding may cease in some patients with diverticular sources following this procedure. Surgery generally is not indicated until 4–6 units of blood have been shed. Coagulation products are of no use unless the patient has abnormal clotting studies. Saline lavage of the colon is not a routine procedure.

17. The answer is B. Many diseases manifest atypically in elderly patients. For example, the presentation, identification, course, and prognosis of peptic ulcer disease may be significantly different in older patients than in younger patients. In the elderly, anorexia and weight loss may be the only presenting symptoms of peptic ulcer disease. Perforation may present without pain and may occur with no prior history of the disease. As in younger patients, tobacco smoking increases the risk of peptic ulcer disease. Giant ulcers occur more commonly in the stomach than in the duodenum.

18. The answer is E. This patient presents with findings and symptoms that are strongly suggestive of acute diverticulitis. Barium enema is contraindicated in this setting due to the possibility of rupturing the abscess into the peritoneum. The most appropriate management would begin with bowel rest (i.e., intravenous fluids and nasogastric suction) and antibiotics. Multiple antibiotic regimens are acceptable; the choice of drugs should be tailored to the usual colonic bacterial flora (i.e., anaerobic organisms and aerobic gram-negative organisms).

19. The answer is D. At this point, the findings in this patient are consistent with a pelvic abscess due to diverticulitis. The pyuria in this situation is due to the proximity of the inflammatory mass to the bladder. Prostatitis presents as pyuria and tenderness of the gland itself, not tenderness in adjacent tissues. Bacteriuria also may be seen in prostatitis. Although diverticulitis is a potential explanation for this syndrome, diverticulosis itself is not an inflammatory condition and does not sufficiently explain these findings. Renal tuberculosis also may be characterized by sterile pyuria; however, this diagnosis does not fit the clinical situation. Urine culture would not help with the diagnosis of diverticular abscess and would not be needed to distinguish prostatitis from an abscess in this situation.

20–23. The answers are: 20-T, 21-F, 22-T, 23-T. Ischemic colitis is most severe where the arterial blood supply to the colon is most limited (i.e., the splenic flexure) and least severe where the blood supply is richest (i.e., the rectum and sigmoid colon). The symptoms are nonspecific and include bloody diarrhea, lower abdominal pain and distension, and occasional vomiting. Diagnosis is suggested by negative findings for other causes of bloody diarrhea (e.g., infection, carcinoma, diverticulosis, angiodysplasia). Also, diverticulosis and angiodysplasia are two causes of bloody diarrhea that typically are painless. Barium enema may show thumb-printing, which represents submucosal edema and hemorrhage.

24–27. The answers are: 24-T, 25-T, 26-T, 27-F. Although endoscopy and biopsy are required to confirm that a gastric ulcer is either benign or malignant, an upper gastrointestinal series can provide useful diagnostic information. Since a malignant ulcer typically occurs in the middle of a gastric mass, the ulcer crater does not extend outside the gastric wall, the folds cannot radiate all the way to the ulcer base, and there is no edema of the surrounding mucosa. The gastric wall is pliable and normally distensible in the area of a benign gastric ulcer, not stiff as with malignant ulcers. In addition, benign ulcers tend to be smooth and round, whereas malignant ulcers are irregular in shape.

28–31. The answers are: 28-F, 29-F, 30-T, 31-F. Diverticulosis and colonic angiodysplasia are equally likely to cause painless massive hematochezia, although rectal hemorrhoids or fissures would be more likely causes if the bleeding were less brisk. Barium enema can establish whether diverticula are present but cannot identify that they are bleeding. This study has been proposed as a therapeutic measure because diverticular bleeding often ceases following the procedure. If the bleeding stops, sigmoidoscopy should be performed first to exclude rectal and sigmoid colonic lesions. If bleeding cannot be controlled, visceral angiography is the procedure of choice to identify the bleeding site. Although rebleeding from diverticular disease occurs, the majority of patients will not experience a second episode.

32–35. The answers are: 32-F, 33-T, 34-F, 35-T. Although adenomatous polyps of the colon are benign, they are considered to be precursors of adenocarcinoma. Size and histology are good determinants of risk for malignancy in these lesions. The risk for adenocarcinoma increases from about 1% in polyps that are smaller than 1 cm to about 50% in those that are larger than 2 cm. In addition, the greatest risk for malignancy is noted in adenomatous polyps that are villous (not tubular) and sessile (not pedunculated). Location within the colon is not a factor in predicting malignancy. If malignancy is present but is confined to the mucosa, localization and removal of the polyp (polypectomy) is curative.

36–39. The answers are: 36-F, 37-T, 38-T, 39-F. The incidence of peptic ulcer disease complications rises considerably with age. The most common complication is bleeding from peptic ulcer disease—a life-threatening emergency that accounts for more than half of all deaths caused by this disease. In treating a patient with a bleeding ulcer, the first priority is restoration of blood pressure and intravenous fluid replacement. Only after these steps have been taken is the bleeding site localized. Although most patients respond to medical therapy alone, recurrent bleeding occurs in up to 30% of patients successfully treated for previous hemorrhage. The mortality rate is increased in older patients, in patients with arteriosclerotic vascular disease, and in gastric versus duodenal ulcers.

40–43. The answers are: 40-T, 41-F, 42-F, 43-T. With advancing age, chronic inflammation of the stomach may progress to atrophic changes in the gastric mucosa—a condition known as atrophic gastritis. Atrophic gastritis is classified as type A or type B, on the basis of distinguishing pathologic and clinical characteristics.

Type B atrophic gastritis is associated with chronic blood loss and with ulceration and atrophy of the gastric mucosa, which are especially marked in the antrum. Gastric acid secretion is reduced somewhat in some patients, but gastrin levels are normal and malabsorption of vitamin B_{12} is rare. Iron deficiency anemia may result, however, due to a reduction of iron absorption. Type B disease rarely is associated with an autoimmune mechanism or other autoimmune diseases.

In contrast, type A atrophic gastritis is associated with mucosal atrophy of the corpus and fundus, with relative sparing of the antrum. Marked achlorhydria is common as is deficiency of intrinsic factor, which leads to malabsorption of vitamin B_{12} and consequent pernicious anemia in these patients. Antibody to parietal cells characteristically is found in the serum of patients with type A disease, and there is a common association with other autoimmune diseases, such as thyroiditis.

44–47. The answers are: 44-T, 45-F, 46-T, 47-T. Colonic diverticula are herniations of the mucosa through the muscularis in areas traversed by vessels. The exact mechanism of diverticular formation is not certain, but several age-related changes in the colon are believed to contribute to the pathogenesis. Primarily, the herniation of colonic mucosa is thought to occur due to structural defects in the muscularis combined with an increase in intraluminal pressure. Chemical changes in the structure of collagen fibers are known to occur with age and are responsible for a thickened muscularis that is less compliant and less resistant to distension. With overdistension of the colonic wall (e.g., due to increased tonic or spasmodic contractions or excessive gas formation), there is an increased pressure gradient between the colonic lumen and the peritoneal cavity and, thus, a risk of herniation. Colonic hypermotility (tonic or spasmodic contractions) in the affected segments of the colon is believed to be caused by age-related degeneration of neurons in the enteric nervous system or lifelong irritable bowel syndrome.

48–51. The answers are: 48-T, 49-F, 50-T, 51-T. Symptoms of gallbladder disease in the elderly often are vague; patients may have poorly localized abdominal pain, minimal fever, and only rarely jaundice. Because of this subtle presentation, the diagnosis of acute cholecystitis may be delayed in older patients, allowing complications (e.g., gangrene, perforation) to occur more frequently than in younger patients.

The diagnosis of acute cholecystitis depends on demonstration of gallstones or nonvisualization of the gallbladder. Abdominal ultrasonography is indicated in the detection of gallstones and is preferred for the diagnosis of acute cholecystitis over oral cholecystography, which is less reliable and requires 24–48 hours to perform.

If surgery is not contraindicated, the therapy of choice is cholecystectomy after resolution of the acute inflammation. A delay of longer than 2 months after the acute phase often results in recurrence of even more severe infection and a higher risk of death. Because of the greater incidence of common bile duct stones in the elderly, choledochotomy often is performed with cholecystectomy in patients who are not at risk for surgery.

3
Respiratory Disorders

QUESTIONS

Directions: Each question below contains five suggested answers. Choose the **one best** response to each question.

1. All of the following drugs are known to cause acute interstitial pneumonitis EXCEPT

(A) hydrochlorothiazide
(B) nitrofurantoin
(C) methotrexate
(D) gold
(E) sulindac

2. Which of the following groups of people is most in need of yearly influenza vaccination?

(A) Residents of nursing homes
(B) Medical personnel who have extensive contact with high-risk groups
(C) Adults with chronic renal failure
(D) Immunosuppressed adults
(E) Adults with chronic disease severe enough to require ongoing medical care

3. An elderly man has been treated for an acute pneumonia with penicillin and then a cephalosporin. He becomes more toxic, however, with fever, pleuritic chest pain, abdominal pain, and confusion. Which organism is the most likely cause of this man's illness?

(A) *Hemophilus influenzae*
(B) *Diplococcus pneumoniae*
(C) *Legionella pneumophila*
(D) *Mycoplasma pneumoniae*
(E) *Mycobacterium tuberculosis*

4. The most effective means of reducing mucous secretions in geriatric patients with coexisting chronic bronchitis and emphysema is with

(A) appropriate antibiotic coverage
(B) a bronchodilator
(C) an expectorant
(D) avoidance of dusty or polluted air
(E) adequate bronchial hydration

5. Which of the following clinical findings is most suggestive of pulmonary embolism in an elderly person with pleuritic chest pain?

(A) Chest wall tenderness
(B) Loud pulmonary component of S_2
(C) New atrial fibrillation
(D) Wheezing and expiratory prolongation
(E) Evidence of deep venous thrombosis

6. A 75-year-old woman who lives in a nursing home where another person was just found to have active pulmonary tuberculosis is admitted to the hospital with a temperature of 102° F, shortness of breath, and chest pain; chest x-ray shows a left lower lobe infiltrate. Initial antibiotic therapy for this patient is best based on

(A) x-ray appearance
(B) Gram stain of sputum
(C) sputum culture results
(D) possible tuberculosis exposure
(E) empiric therapy (to include coverage for gram-negative organisms)

7. COPD is a common cause of pulmonary hypertension in the elderly. The most potent stimulus for the development of pulmonary hypertension in COPD is

(A) hypercapnia
(B) alveolar membrane damage
(C) left ventricular failure
(D) hypoxia
(E) acidosis

8. The most common cause of sporadic pneumonia in the elderly is

(A) *Mycoplasma pneumoniae*
(B) *Streptococcus pneumoniae*
(C) *Staphylococcus aureus*
(D) *Hemophilus influenzae*
(E) *Legionella pneumophila*

9. An elderly man has been hospitalized for 1 week because of severe and worsening Parkinson's disease. He is found in bed tachypneic, tachycardic, and responsive only to painful stimuli. Pulmonary examination reveals diffuse rhonchi and rales in the right lung field posteriorly and absent breath sounds in the left. Which of the following conditions is most likely to be responsible for this patient's presentation?

(A) Massive pulmonary embolism
(B) Pulmonary edema after acute myocardial infarction
(C) Aspiration pneumonia with unilateral bronchial obstruction
(D) Spontaneous pneumothorax
(E) Tracheoesophageal fistula

10. An elderly patient is seriously ill with pneumonia. The etiology is unclear and the Gram stain of sputum is not helpful. Initial antibiotic coverage is best provided with

(A) penicillin alone
(B) a first-generation cephalosporin
(C) penicillin plus doxycycline
(D) erythromycin plus an aminoglycoside
(E) no treatment until the etiologic agent is positively identified on sputum culture

11. Which of the following statements best characterizes asthma as it occurs in the elderly population?

(A) Asthma usually is of the allergic type
(B) Acute attacks often are precipitated by viral respiratory infection
(C) The clinical presentation typically includes episodic wheezing and dyspnea, just as in younger patients
(D) Serum IgE levels and blood eosinophil counts usually are elevated
(E) Subcutaneous epinephrine is a standard treatment

Questions 12–14

A 71-year-old man who smokes is hospitalized for thrombophlebitis for the second time in 8 months. The patient has had no pulmonary symptoms and otherwise is in good health, but chest x-ray reveals a solitary peripheral nodule in the right lower lobe.

12. Initial evaluation of this patient should include all of the following items EXCEPT

(A) reviewing previous chest x-rays
(B) obtaining a travel history
(C) bronchoscopy
(D) tuberculosis skin testing
(E) sputum cytology

13. Tomography ordered in the evaluation of this patient demonstrates a lesion in the distal periphery of the left lower lobe, with ill-defined margins and no calcifications. Other results of the initial evaluation are not helpful. What is the best course of action at this time?

(A) Repeat chest x-ray in 4 months
(B) Treatment with isoniazid
(C) Culture sputum for tuberculosis
(D) Radiation therapy
(E) Thoracotomy

14. A squamous cell carcinoma ultimately is removed from this patient after negative metastatic workup. All biopsied nodes are negative for metastasis. However, 18 months after removal of the lesion, another single pulmonary nodule is noted in the periphery of the right lung. Repeat metastatic workup is negative, and pulmonary function testing reveals findings of mild to moderate COPD. What is the best course of action now?

(A) Repeat chest x-ray in 4 months
(B) Chemotherapy
(C) Radiation therapy
(D) A second thoracotomy
(E) No further interventions can be offered

Directions: The groups of questions below consist of an introductory premise or case data followed by four statements that pertain to the information given. Indicate whether each statement is **true** or **false**.

Questions 15–18

The following statements accurately describe the polyvalent pneumococcal vaccine.

15. The pneumococcal vaccine should not be given on the same visit as influenza vaccination

16. Pneumococcal vaccination should be given yearly

17. Very elderly patients exhibit impaired antibody responses to the pneumococcal vaccine

18. When vaccinated nursing home residents develop pneumococcal pneumonia, the illness usually is caused by serotypes not included in the vaccine

Questions 19–22

Pulmonary function is affected by several age-related changes in the respiratory system. The following factors change with age.

19. Lung compliance

20. Alveolar–arterial PO_2 gradient

21. Arterial PCO_2

22. Pulmonary vascular resistance during exercise

Questions 23–26

A 60-year-old woman with moderately advanced COPD and mild wheezing requires an exploratory laparotomy. The following preoperative measures can reduce postoperative complications.

23. Corticosteroid administration

24. Instruction in "pulmonary toilet"

25. Discontinuance of cigarette smoking

26. Use of a bronchodilator such as aminophylline

Questions 27–30

Pulmonary embolism is suspected in a 70-year-old woman with pleuritic chest pain and shortness of breath. Pulmonary angiography should be the next test performed in the following situations for the diagnosis of pulmonary embolism.

27. Normal arterial blood gas analysis, including a normal alveolar–arterial PO_2 gradient

28. An increased alveolar–arterial PO_2 gradient with a subsegmental defect on perfusion scanning

29. An abnormal venogram performed for leg swelling

30. An abnormal chest x-ray with a Hampton's hump

Questions 31–34

The risk for developing active tuberculosis is much higher in elderly persons than in the general population. The following statements describe this infection as it occurs in the elderly.

31. Tuberculosis usually results from reactivation of a primary infection that occurred earlier in life

32. Most cases of tuberculosis are associated with reactivity to tuberculin skin tests

33. Tuberculosis usually is an extrapulmonary infection

34. When pulmonary infection is present, it usually is associated with a pleural effusion

Questions 35–38

The following organisms commonly are responsible for lower respiratory tract infections in patients with COPD.

35. *Branhamella catarrhalis*

36. *Streptococcus pneumoniae*

37. *Hemophilus influenzae*

38. *Pseudomonas aeruginosa*

Questions 39–42

In addition to cigarette smoking, factors that are associated with the development of emphysema include the following.

39. Cadmium exposure

40. Heterozygous α_1-antitrypsin deficiency

41. Air pollution

42. Bronchial asthma

Questions 43–46

Theophylline, a bronchodilator used extensively for COPD, may accumulate to toxic levels as a result of coexisting illness or concomitantly administered drugs in geriatric patients. The following factors can result in elevated theophylline levels.

43. Heavy smoking

44. Hepatic cirrhosis

45. Treatment with penicillin

46. Treatment with cimetidine

Questions 47–50

A 62-year-old woman who has congestive heart failure develops pneumonia and a large pleural effusion. Thoracentesis is performed in an effort to establish the etiology of the pleural effusion (i.e., congestive heart failure or pneumonia). The following pleural fluid findings would indicate that the pleural effusion is due to congestive heart failure.

47. A protein content of 6 g/dl

48. A pH of 7.13

49. A glucose content of 20 mg/dl

50. An LDH content of 100 mg/dl (with a serum LDH level of 420 mg/dl)

ANSWERS AND EXPLANATIONS

1. The answer is E. Many drugs may accumulate in the lungs and cause acute or chronic injury. Certain drugs (e.g., hydrochlorothiazide, nitrofurantoin, methotrexate, gold) are responsible for an acute interstitial pneumonitis; this disease typically presents as dyspnea, fever, and bilateral interstitial infiltrates on chest x-ray. Other agents (e.g., bleomycin, phenytoin) cause changes that occur with diffuse end-stage pulmonary fibrosis. Sulindac has not been implicated in either of these forms of drug-induced pulmonary disease.

2. The answer is A. Residents of nursing homes are at highest risk for developing influenza during epidemics, with attack rates of 60% and fatality rates approaching 30%. Adults who are immunosuppressed, adults with chronic renal failure or some other chronic disorder that requires continuous medical care, and medical personnel who have extensive exposure to high-risk groups also should receive the vaccine, but the priority is lower for these population groups.

3. The answer is C. *Legionella pneumophila* always should be suspected as the cause of a pneumonic process that does not respond to initial therapy, especially in the presence of gastrointestinal and CNS symptoms. Diplococcal pneumonia should respond to both penicillin and cephalosporins, and pneumonia due to *Hemophilus influenzae* should respond to a cephalosporin. *Mycoplasma pneumoniae* would be unusual in this age-group and probably would not cause such severe illness. The onset of tuberculosis usually is over days to weeks, with low-grade fever, night sweats, and weight loss.

4. The answer is D. Chronic bronchitis and emphysema are components of COPD—a common pulmonary disorder usually characterized by progressive obstruction to airflow and a history of inhalation of irritants. Cigarette smoking is the primary etiologic agent; polluted air contributes to the damage done by smoking. The most effective management of patients with COPD is avoidance of exposure to these irritants. Patients should be advised to stop smoking, to stay indoors during times of heavy air pollution, and to avoid dusty or smoky areas. Other means of reducing or facilitating removal of mucous secretions in these patients include bronchial hydration, mucolytic agents, expectorants, bronchodilators, and antibiotics. Some of these treatments are costly, however, and may cause adverse effects. Therefore, removal of the primary irritants, if possible, is the best management.

5. The answer is E. Pulmonary embolism may have a subtle presentation, with somewhat nonspecific clinical features that may be missed in elderly patients (i.e., patients may be thought to have pneumonia). Symptoms include hyperventilation, faintness or syncope, dyspnea, pleuritic chest pain, cough, and hemoptysis. Physical examination suggests the presence of deep venous thrombosis in 50% of patients with pulmonary embolism. Since physical findings in deep venous thrombosis may be seen in other disorders (e.g., cellulitis, popliteal cyst), venography or noninvasive testing must be performed to confirm clinical suspicion. Other findings may include a pleuritic friction rub, percussion dullness, and decreased breath sounds. Although a loud pulmonary component of S_2 may be noted, this is a nonspecific finding. Wheezing and expiratory prolongation also are nonspecific findings that are seen more typically in COPD than in pulmonary embolism. Although a new arrhythmia may be a manifestation of pulmonary embolism, it is a nonspecific finding and atrial fibrillation would not be the most likely rhythm disturbance. Chest wall tenderness is not a clinical component of pulmonary embolism.

6. The answer is B. The initial selection of an antibiotic for treatment of a pulmonary infection is best based on the Gram stain of an adequate sputum specimen. Radiographic appearance is useful for predicting likely causative organisms (e.g., "typical" lobar pneumonia is likely bacterial, whereas patchy and bilateral infiltrates suggest "atypical" pneumonia due to *Mycoplasma pneumoniae*, a virus, or *Legionella pneumophila*). Sputum culture results usually are not available until after 48 hours; further, *Streptococcus pneumoniae* may not grow on culture media and must be seen on Gram stain for diagnosis. Tuberculosis exposure must be considered and appropriate sputum samples collected for AFB smear and cultures, but this patient presents with a syndrome more typical of a bacterial infection and initially should be treated for one. Respiratory isolation precaution may be appropriate until smear results are known to be negative. Although persons living in nursing homes resemble hospitalized patients in that they often are colonized by gram-negative organisms, empiric therapy is the best approach only when adequate sputum samples cannot be obtained.

7. The answer is D. Pulmonary hypertension in elderly patients with COPD is due primarily to the vasoconstrictive effect of hypoxia. This response may be increased by acidosis, which also has a direct, although less dramatic, vasoconstrictive effect on the pulmonary vasculature. Hypercapnia also can contribute to pulmonary vasoconstriction, probably via local acidosis. Pulmonary vasoconstriction puts a strain on the right ventricle, leading to its eventual failure (cor pulmonale). Left ventricular failure occurs independently of right ventricular failure and usually is caused by atherosclerotic coronary artery disease or hypertension. In patients with emphysema, a loss of the pulmonary capillary bed is the underlying factor predisposing to pulmonary hypertension.

8. The answer is B. *Streptococcus pneumoniae* remains the most common cause of sporadic bacterial pneumonia in the elderly; although *Hemophilus influenzae* is a frequent agent of pneumonia in this age-group, it is implicated less often than *S. pneumoniae*. *Staphylococcus aureus* and gram-negative organisms are the most frequent causes of nosocomial bacterial pneumonia. *Mycoplasma pneumoniae* is the most common agent of atypical community-acquired pneumonia in younger adults. Elderly persons rarely are affected by *M. pneumoniae*; *Legionella pneumophila* and viruses are the most frequent agents implicated in this syndrome in geriatric patients.

9. The answer is C. The most likely cause of this patient's presentation is aspiration pneumonia with unilateral large bronchial obstruction. Patients with severe Parkinson's disease are predisposed to aspiration because of problems with swallowing, and large-airway obstruction on the left could occur concomitantly with a pneumonic process on the right. Pulmonary embolism typically does not cause such abnormalities on pulmonary examination, although an immobile patient with Parkinson's disease would be at an increased risk for this problem because of a greater risk for associated venous thrombosis. Pulmonary edema also is not typically associated with such unusual findings on lung examination. Spontaneous pneumothorax is a more likely event in younger patients or those with COPD and is unlikely to produce the right lung findings seen in this patient. Patients with tracheoesophageal fistula can present with recurrent aspiration pneumonia, but there is no reason to suspect that abnormality in this patient.

10. The answer is D. The seriousness of infection in this patient demands that antibiotic coverage be broad and aggressive from the onset of therapy; the physiologic reserve in a seriously ill elderly patient may not allow time for errors in antibiotic coverage. If the clinical or radiographic appearance is "atypical," empiric therapy should include erythromycin or other drugs effective against *Legionella pneumophila*—the most dangerous pathogenic agent of atypical community-acquired pneumonia in the elderly.

11. The answer is B. Asthma is a disease characterized by hyperirritability of the airways; substances that have no effect when inhaled by normal persons cause bronchoconstriction in asthmatic persons. Asthma often is classified as allergic or nonallergic. The allergic type is responsible for most cases of childhood asthma; the nonallergic type accounts for most cases in adults, including the elderly. Other pathogenetic and clinical features characterize asthma in elderly patients. Most acute episodes are precipitated by a respiratory infection, typically due to a virus or *Mycoplasma*. Wheezing and dyspnea, which are episodic and regarded as classic symptoms in younger patients, often are continuous in older patients; moreover, it is important to consider other causes of such symptoms in geriatric patients (e.g., congestive heart failure). Serum IgE levels are variable, and blood eosinophil counts may be normal in elderly patients with nonallergic asthma. Subcutaneous epinephrine should not be used to treat elderly asthmatics due to its potential for causing arrhythmias, negative hemodynamic effects, and tachyphylaxis. Methylxanthine preparations or more selective β-adrenergic agonists are the standard treatment in these patients. Inhaled anticholinergic agents are increasingly being used in these patients (e.g., ipratropium).

12. The answer is C. Bronchoscopy is not typically part of the initial evaluation and is unlikely to be helpful in evaluating a peripheral lesion. Previous chest x-rays may show that the lesion has not grown in recent years, thus suggesting a benign lesion. A recent travel history (e.g., to the San Joaquin Valley for a diagnosis of primary coccidioidomycosis, or "valley fever") may be useful. Skin testing for tuberculosis would provide useful additional information to direct other diagnostic efforts, and if sputum cytology proved the presence of a malignancy, treatment decisions then could be made.

13. The answer is E. A thoracotomy is indicated for this patient's pulmonary lesion. An older patient with a pulmonary nodule that is less than 1.5 cm and does not contain calcium should be treated surgically, if that patient is a good candidate for surgery. Although percutaneous transthoracic needle biopsy is a feasible procedure in this setting, thoracotomy generally is preferred for a newly diagnosed distal coin lesion, since the diagnosis and treatment can be coupled. Further, a histologic diagnosis often is impossible by needle biopsy, although the presence or absence of cancer usually can be ascertained.

14. The answer is D. The data available suggest that this patient has another primary pulmonary malignancy and should be treated for such (with thoracotomy), as long as a second operation can be tolerated. Even with mild to moderate COPD, this patient most likely can tolerate a second lobar resection, which may be curative.

15–18. The answers are: 15-F, 16-F, 17-T, 18-T. The polyvalent pneumococcal vaccine probably is 60%–80% efficacious in preventing pneumococcal disease in the elderly when the illness is caused by 1 of the 23 strains whose capsular polysaccharides are contained in the vaccine. It can be given at a different injection site on the same visit that the influenza vaccine is administered. The pneumococcal vaccine has a very low incidence of systemic adverse reactions; but these are more common when patients are revaccinated, and additional doses usually give poor "booster" effects. Present guidelines suggest vaccination only once in a lifetime, even though very elderly patients exhibit marked decline in antibody levels 1 year after immunization. One report has suggested that as many as 70% of cases of pneumococcal pneumonia in vaccinated persons are caused by serotypes not included in the vaccine; however, the overall frequency of pneumococcal pneumonia is decreased.

19–22. The answers are: 19-T, 20-T, 21-F, 22-T. The change in volume per unit change in pressure (lung compliance) during spontaneous breathing increases with age. Reduced elastic recoil of the lungs accounts for this increased compliance. Increased rigidity of the chest wall with aging, however, nearly compensates for increased lung expandability. Because arterial PO_2 declines with age, the alveolar–arterial PO_2 gradient also increases. Although pulmonary vascular resistance is unchanged during resting conditions, it increases during exercise, presumably as a result of reduced elasticity and narrowing of the pulmonary arteries. Arterial PCO_2 does not change with age.

23–26. The answers are: 23-F, 24-T, 25-T, 26-T. Certain pre- and postoperative measures can improve pulmonary function and reduce the number of postoperative complications. Preoperative instruction in the methods of "pulmonary toilet" to be used postoperatively is helpful to ensure patient compliance. Cigarette smoking should be stopped at least 2–3 weeks preceding surgery to eliminate the acute effects of smoking on the respiratory epithelium, but smoking cessation even 1 or 2 days prior to surgery may be helpful. To some degree, bronchodilators can improve wheezing in patients with lung disease. Steroids should be avoided before surgery because of their association with impaired wound healing and decreased resistance to infection.

27–30. The answers are: 27-F, 28-T, 29-F, 30-F. Pulmonary angiography is the standard test for definitive diagnosis of pulmonary embolism. However, when ventilation and perfusion scanning, arterial blood gas analysis, or both produce perfectly normal results and the alveolar–arterial PO_2 gradient is normal, pulmonary embolism is extremely unlikely.

In most patients, totally normal arterial blood gases and a normal alveolar–arterial PO_2 gradient would be sufficient evidence to exclude pulmonary embolism. If suspicion were still high, ventilation and perfusion scanning should be the next step.

Several conditions can cause subsegmental scanning defects and an abnormal alveolar–arterial PO_2 gradient; therefore, pulmonary angiography should be performed in such situations because these tests neither confirm nor exclude pulmonary embolism.

An abnormal venogram is sufficient evidence to begin anticoagulant therapy in this patient. However, ventilation and perfusion scanning should be performed to provide better evidence for pulmonary embolism.

A Hampton's hump (i.e., a nodular density at the costophrenic angle, seen on chest x-ray) suggests pulmonary embolism with infarction. Although pulmonary angiography could be performed for definitive diagnosis, ventilation and perfusion scanning is safer and would typically be performed before angiography in this setting.

31–34. The answers are: 31-T, 32-T, 33-F, 34-F. Reactivation of an earlier primary infection remains the most common origin of clinical tuberculosis in the elderly. In many cases, however, epidemics in nursing homes are associated with primary inoculation, such that new infection is becoming more common in this group of patients. About 80% of patients with reactivation tuberculosis react to intermediate-strength PPD testing, although malnutrition, widespread disease, and very old age predispose to a higher percentage of anergy. Although extrapulmonary infection without clinical evidence of tuberculous pulmonary disease is becoming more common, tuberculosis is predominantly a pulmonary disease in the elderly. Pleural effusion is not a common feature of pulmonary tuberculosis in these patients; pleural reaction typically is a manifestation of primary infections, although in rare cases it can occur when an established lung focus extends to the pleural space.

35–38. The answers are: 35-F, 36-T, 37-T, 38-F. *Branhamella catarrhalis*, *Streptococcus pneumoniae*, and *Hemophilus influenzae* commonly colonize the upper and lower respiratory tract of patients with COPD, and *S. pneumoniae* and *H. influenzae* have long been known to be common causes of bacterial bronchitis and pneumonia in these patients. Recently, *B. catarrhalis* also has been described as a potential cause of bronchitis and pneumonia in COPD patients, but it is an uncommon cause of such infections. In a patient with a pulmonary infection who is found to have *B. catarrhalis* on sputum culture, the best initial antibiotic choice would be erythromycin or trimethoprim-sulfamethoxazole, since 40% of these bacteria produce β lactamase and, thus, would not be sensitive to penicillin (used to treat *S. pneumoniae*) or ampicillin (used to treat *H. influenzae*). *Pseudomonas aeruginosa* would be a common cause of lower respiratory tract infections only in seriously ill patients already on antibiotics or a ventilator.

39–42. The answers are: 39-T, 40-F, 41-T, 42-F. Although the exact cause of emphysema is unknown, several factors are known to contribute to its development. Cigarette smoking is the most important factor predisposing to obstructive emphysema. In addition, certain types of environmental exposure correlate with an increased incidence of emphysema. Examples include occupational exposure to cadmium fumes (cadmium also is a component of cigarette fumes) and chronic exposure to industrial air pollution. Homozygous α_1-antitrypsin deficiency is another risk factor, which has been associated with panlobular emphysema; this association does not exist with heterozygous α_1-antitrypsin deficiency. Some studies suggest that the heterozygous state is a cofactor with cigarette smoking for centrilobular emphysema, but this hypothesis is not yet widely accepted. Bronchial asthma may cause a temporary obstructive picture and even pulmonary hypertension in the acute episode, but it rarely is implicated as a cause of emphysema.

43–46. The answers are: 43-F, 44-T, 45-F, 46-T. Theophylline is a potent bronchodilating agent that is used in the treatment of COPD. It is eliminated primarily by metabolism in the liver; only about 10% of administered theophylline exists unchanged in the urine. Hepatic dysfunction may significantly decrease the clearance of theophylline and result in toxic concentrations in the plasma. For example, in patients with hepatic cirrhosis, the effect of decreased clearance causes the plasma half-life of theophylline to increase from a normal value of 8 or 9 hours to as high as 60 hours. Concomitant use of certain drugs, such as cimetidine and erythromycin, also causes a decreased clearance of theophylline. In contrast, certain other drugs appear to increase the metabolism of theophylline. Nicotine and phenytoin are examples of such agents. Penicillin is not known to affect the disposition of theophylline.

47–50. The answers are: 47-F, 48-F, 49-F, 50-T. In establishing the etiology of a pleural effusion, it is useful to determine whether the fluid is a transudate or an exudate. This determination often can be made on the basis of a chemical analysis of the pleural fluid. A pleural fluid protein content of more than 3 g/dl and an LDH content of more than 250 mg/dl usually indicate the presence of an exudate. In addition, an exudate usually is associated with a pleural fluid-to-serum protein ratio of less than 0.5 and a pleural fluid-to-serum LDH ratio of less than 0.6. Pleural fluid pH values below 7.2 and a pleural fluid glucose content of less than 20 mg/dl also are associated with inflammatory effusions (exudates). With the exception of the LDH findings, all of the pleural fluid findings listed indicate the presence of an exudate. Exudates are caused by inflammation or disease of the pleural surface or by lymphatic obstruction (e.g., due to tuberculosis, lung cancer, or pneumonia). Transudates are caused by elevated systemic or pulmonary venous pressure or by decreased plasma oncotic pressure (e.g., due to congestive heart failure or nephrotic syndrome).

4
Cardiovascular Disorders

QUESTIONS

Directions: Each question below contains five suggested answers. Choose the **one best** response to each question.

1. According to the Framingham study, significant risk factors for cardiovascular mortality in men between 65 and 74 years of age include all of the following EXCEPT

(A) hypertension
(B) cigarette smoking
(C) serum cholesterol level
(D) proteinuria
(E) electrocardiographic evidence of left ventricular hypertrophy

2. Which of the following statements is true regarding cardiovascular function and the normal process of aging?

(A) Cardiac muscle loses the ability to develop tension
(B) Cardiac muscle has a decreased inotropic response to calcium
(C) Cardiac muscle has a decreased inotropic response to catecholamines
(D) Left ventricular function at rest is decreased
(E) The Frank-Starling mechanism is less effective in compensating for the demands of exercise

3. The most frequent type of valvular heart disease in the elderly is

(A) pulmonic stenosis
(B) mitral stenosis
(C) mitral regurgitation
(D) aortic stenosis
(E) aortic regurgitation

4. The potent, positive inotropic effect of digoxin makes it an important drug for the treatment of congestive heart failure. All of the following statements regarding digoxin are true EXCEPT

(A) the dosage should be reduced in patients receiving quinidine
(B) severe toxicity is treated best with dialysis
(C) toxicity may occur at apparently therapeutic serum levels
(D) to monitor serum levels, blood should be drawn 6–8 hours after the last dose
(E) elderly patients are prone to toxic neurologic effects of digoxin

5. Embolic arterial disease is encountered with increasing frequency in the elderly population. All of the following statements regarding arterial embolism in elderly patients are true EXCEPT

(A) rheumatic heart disease is an etiologic factor in relatively few cases of arterial embolism
(B) the left atrium and left ventricle are common sources of emboli
(C) the aorta is an unusual source of emboli
(D) numbness and paresthesias may be the initial symptoms of arterial embolism
(E) an embolus in the popliteal artery should be treated conservatively rather than with embolectomy

6. All of the following conduction abnormalities are accepted indications for permanent pacemaker placement EXCEPT

(A) asymptomatic complete heart block with ventricular ectopy
(B) complete heart block with congestive heart failure
(C) complete heart block that persists after an anterior myocardial infarction
(D) syncope, in which a cardiovascular cause is suspected but the ECG is normal
(E) symptomatic sick sinus syndrome

7. Common causes of mitral valve defects in elderly patients include all of the following disorders EXCEPT

(A) rheumatic heart disease
(B) rheumatoid arthritis
(C) papillary muscle dysfunction
(D) mitral annulus calcification
(E) myxomatous degeneration of the mitral valve cusps

8. A 75-year-old man is admitted to the hospital complaining of fatigue, dyspnea on exertion, orthopnea, and swollen feet. The clinical evaluation reveals the following findings: blood pressure of 90/60 mm Hg, regular pulse of 100/min, neck vein distension with central venous pressure estimated at 12 cm H_2O, a systolic ejection murmur that radiates to the neck, a markedly delayed carotid upstroke, bibasilar pulmonary rales, and 2+ peripheral edema. All of the following statements concerning this case are true EXCEPT

(A) a diagnostic workup for the cause of the patient's heart failure is indicated
(B) the patient has evidence of biventricular failure
(C) increased afterload is a likely mechanism for the patient's left ventricular heart failure
(D) diuretic therapy may ameliorate the patient's orthopnea and edema
(E) afterload reduction therapy with captopril should be employed

9. Antiarrhythmic therapy is required for all of the elderly patients described below EXCEPT

(A) a 70-year-old man with recurrent sustained ventricular tachycardia
(B) an 82-year-old man with more than 30 ventricular premature beats/hr and occasional couplets
(C) a 78-year-old woman who has recently experienced ventricular fibrillation
(D) a 72-year-old woman on no medications with an episode of *torsades de pointes* in the setting of a long QT interval on ECG
(E) a 75-year-old man with an ejection fraction less than 40% and complex ventricular ectopy

10. Blood pressure tends to rise with age. In addition, the stiffening of arteries with advancing age causes a disproportionate increase in systolic blood pressure. The initial evaluation of an elderly patient with isolated systolic hypertension requires all of the following studies EXCEPT

(A) serum creatinine measurement
(B) serum glucose measurement
(C) serum potassium measurement
(D) urinalysis
(E) echocardiography

11. Which of the following vasodilating agents acts solely by reducing preload?

(A) Hydralazine
(B) Nifedipine
(C) Nitroglycerin
(D) Captopril
(E) Prazosin

12. The cardiovascular response to exercise in a healthy elderly person is different from the response in a younger adult in all of the following ways EXCEPT

(A) a lower heart rate response occurs at each work load level
(B) a lesser increase in stroke volume occurs for a given cardiac output
(C) the end-systolic volume is larger
(D) the end-diastolic volume is larger
(E) the ejection fraction increases to a lesser extent

13. Sick sinus syndrome is primarily a disorder of elderly persons. Which of the following statements regarding sick sinus syndrome is true?

(A) Both tachycardia and bradycardia must be present to make the diagnosis
(B) When symptomatic tachycardia is documented, both drug therapy and pacemaker insertion are necessary
(C) A simple ventricular demand (VVI) pacemaker is adequate for most symptomatic patients
(D) Digoxin alone can be used safely in patients with sinus pauses of less than 2 seconds
(E) Quinidine can be used as initial therapy if atrial fibrillation is part of the syndrome

14. Postphlebitic syndrome is associated with all of the following conditions EXCEPT

(A) chronic stasis ulceration
(B) venous valvular incompetence
(C) venous claudication
(D) recurrent pulmonary embolism
(E) dermatitis

Directions: The groups of questions below consist of an introductory premise or case data followed by four statements that pertain to the information given. Indicate whether each statement is **true** or **false**.

Questions 15–18

The clinical presentation of severe aortic stenosis can be subtle; therefore, recognition of physical signs of the disorder is important. The following findings on physical examination are signs of severe aortic stenosis.

15. A harsh, late-peaking systolic ejection murmur

16. A loud aortic component of S_2

17. A delayed carotid upstroke

18. A diastolic rumble

Questions 19–22

The syndrome of myocardial infarction is somewhat different in older patients (over age 70 years) than in younger ones. The following effects of age are noted.

19. Mortality rates are unchanged in older patients

20. The clinical setting is more severe in older patients

21. Ventricular arrhythmias occur more commonly in older patients

22. Cardiac rupture occurs more commonly in older patients

Questions 23–26

The following statements accurately describe the actions and uses of calcium channel blocking agents (verapamil, nifedipine, diltiazem) in patients with cardiovascular disorders.

23. All of the calcium channel blockers act by decreasing preload and increasing afterload

24. Nifedipine is the most useful for treating hypertension

25. Verapamil is particularly effective for treating supraventricular tachycardias

26. Diltiazem is contraindicated in patients with congestive heart failure

Questions 27–30

The following statements accurately describe the clinical presentation and diagnosis of deep venous thrombosis.

27. Impedance plethysmography and Doppler ultrasonography are useful for the diagnosis of thigh thrombi

28. Radiolabeled fibrinogen scanning is useful for the evaluation of calf vein thrombi

29. Calf vein thrombi rarely embolize to the lung

30. Pulmonary embolism is unlikely if lower extremity venography is normal

Questions 31–34

The following statements accurately describe multifocal atrial tachycardia.

31. It is an arrhythmia commonly seen in patients with respiratory failure

32. It commonly is associated with digitalis intoxication

33. It often does not require specific therapy

34. It can be treated with carotid sinus massage

CASE 1: Questions 35–46

Questions 35–38

A 92-year-old man arrives at his physician's office complaining of the sudden onset of lightheadedness, palpitations, and shortness of breath 4 hours prior to his visit. He admits to similar episodes over the previous year, which resolved spontaneously. On examination, the patient is somewhat agitated, with an irregular pulse of 106/min, a blood pressure of 118/75 mm Hg, and a slightly increased respiratory rate. Bibasilar inspiratory crackles are noted, but there is no pedal or sacral edema; the ECG shows new atrial fibrillation. The following measures should be taken in the initial management of this patient.

35. Arterial blood gas analysis

36. Immediate cardioversion

37. Intravenous administration of digoxin

38. Initiation of anticoagulation

Questions 39–42

The patient is stabilized with intravenous digoxin. As his ventricular rate drops below 100 beats/min, he becomes comfortable, although he still is in atrial fibrillation. The following diagnostic studies should be undertaken at this time.

39. Serial serum CK and LDH isoenzyme studies

40. Thyroid function studies

41. Echocardiography

42. Pulmonary angiography

Questions 43–46

After completion of the diagnostic studies listed above, no cause is identified for this patient's arrhythmia. Despite drug treatment, he remains in atrial fibrillation, and the decision is made to try cardioversion. The following statements regarding this procedure are accurate.

43. Cardioversion can be used in the initial management of atrial fibrillation

44. A higher level of energy is required to convert atrial fibrillation than to convert atrial flutter

45. The shorter the duration of the arrhythmia, the more likely that cardioversion will be successful

46. Anticoagulation should precede cardioversion in patients with mitral valve disease and a history of thromboembolism

CASE 2: Questions 47–58

Questions 47–50

A normally healthy 63-year-old man with a history of mild claudication and occasional ulcer symptoms comes to the emergency room after 4 hours of severe midabdominal to epigastric pain and nausea. He denies diaphoresis, chest pain, and shortness of breath. Based on this information, the differential diagnosis should include the following disorders.

47. Perforated viscus

48. Abdominal aortic aneurysm

49. Intestinal angina

50. Myocardial infarction

Questions 51–54

The patient is found to have a pulsatile abdominal mass in the periumbilical area, with a bruit. His vital signs and physical condition have remained stable and unchanged over the past 2 hours. The diagnostic evaluation at this point should include the following procedures.

51. Abdominal ultrasonography

52. Anterior-posterior and lateral abdominal x-rays

53. Abdominal CT scanning

54. Aortography

Questions 55–58

The diagnosis of abdominal aortic aneurysm is made and the size of the aneurysm is determined to be about 5 cm. The following statements address issues that must be considered in the treatment of this patient.

55. Symptoms often portend rupture in a patient with aortic aneurysm

56. The mortality rate for elective resection is drastically lower than that for operation after rupture

57. Small aneurysms may be followed with regular ultrasonography rather than surgery

58. Death after elective surgery usually is due to disorders in other organ systems

ANSWERS AND EXPLANATIONS

1. The answer is C. The risk factors for cardiovascular mortality in the elderly, as identified in the Framingham study, demonstrate differences between men and women. Some factors, such as hypertension, proteinuria, and left ventricular hypertrophy by electrocardiographic criteria (by far the most strongly correlated factor) represent significant risks in both men and women. Diabetes and vital capacity are significant factors only in women, whereas cigarette smoking is significantly related only in men. According to this study, serum cholesterol level and obesity are unrelated to cardiovascular mortality in both men and women in this age-group.

2. The answer is C. Age-related changes in the cardiovascular tissues are more selective than global in nature. Many cardiovascular functions do not decrease with advancing age. For example, the ability of the cardiac muscle to develop tension, left ventricular function at rest, and the inotropic response of cardiac muscle to calcium are unchanged. The response of cardiac muscle to catecholamine stimulation during stress is significantly blunted, however, resulting in decreased inotropic response, decreased arterial dilation, and decreased chronotropic response. In healthy elderly persons, stroke volume is maintained during left ventricular loading by enhanced use of the Frank-Starling mechanism, thus compensating for the decreased cardiovascular response to adrenergic stimulation.

3. The answer is D. Aortic stenosis is the most common form of valvular heart disease in the elderly. In patients between the ages of 50 and 70 years, the most frequent cause of aortic stenosis is calcification of a congenitally bicuspid valve; in those older than 75 years, the most common cause is degenerative calcification of a previously normal aortic valve. Clinically significant aortic stenosis may appear quite rapidly (i.e., within 6–8 months), and recognition of the problem may be complicated by the possible presence of numerous other causes of systolic murmurs. A useful procedure for evaluating significant aortic stenosis is an echocardiogram to look for evidence of aortic valvular calcification as well as decreased mobility and orifice size.

4. The answer is B. Although digoxin therapy often is the cornerstone of pharmacologic treatment of congestive heart failure, it has several drawbacks. Toxicity is a common problem, with the most frequent effects being cardiac arrhythmias, gastrointestinal disorders (e.g., abdominal cramps, diarrhea, vomiting), and CNS disorders (e.g., headache, fatigue, confusion). Elderly patients with atherosclerotic disease are particularly prone to toxic neurologic effects, including disorientation, delirium, and hallucinations. Although routine measurement of serum digoxin concentration is a useful guide, at least 10% of patients have toxic effects when serum levels are within the normal range. To monitor serum digoxin concentration, blood must be drawn at least 6–8 hours after administration of a dose. Drug interactions also can affect serum digoxin level. For example, concomitant use of quinidine can cause the serum concentration of digoxin to double. Digoxin is not dialyzable, but antibodies to digoxin are available for emergency management of extreme toxicity.

5. The answer is E. Arterial embolism is a dangerous situation associated with a relatively high mortality rate due to the advanced age and underlying diseases of most patients who are affected. The most common etiologic factors are atherosclerotic coronary artery disease, recent myocardial infarction, and atrial fibrillation; rheumatic heart disease is less commonly encountered as a cause of arterial embolism in elderly patients. The usual origin of the embolus is the left atrium or left ventricle; much less often, the source is an atheromatous lesion of the aorta. Although the sudden onset of severe pain in a lower extremity is the usual presentation, some patients present with numbness and paresthesias in the absence of initial pain. Embolectomy is indicated for management of emboli that lodge in larger vessels (i.e., the aorta, femoral arteries, or popliteal arteries).

6. The answer is D. Electrocardiographic findings of specific conduction disturbances are the best indications of the need for permanent pacemaker placement. Any symptomatic patient with an arrhythmia must be evaluated, taking into account electrocardiographic findings, symptoms, prognosis, and accompanying medical problems. Persistent complete heart block and symptomatic sick sinus syndrome are indications for permanent pacemaker placement. Complete heart block that occurs in the setting of acute inferior myocardial infarction often reverts to normal sinus rhythm as ischemia of the AV node resolves. Conversely, complete heart block in the setting of anterior myocardial infarction generally implies more widespread ischemia or infarction of the conduction system bundle branches and less often reverts to sinus rhythm. When the ECG is normal and a cardiovascular cause of syncope is suspected, electrophysiologic testing should be performed before permanent pacemaker insertion. Studies are in progress to identify risk factors at other points in the conduction system, particularly the

His-Purkinje system, which may lead to a change in the therapeutic approach to conduction disturbances.

7. The answer is B. Valvular heart disease is common in the geriatric population. Although aortic stenosis is the most common lesion, mitral valve defects also occur frequently. Several disorders can adversely affect the structure and function of the mitral valve. Rheumatic heart disease still is regarded as the major cause of mitral valve dysfunction in the elderly. Although the incidence of rheumatic fever is declining steadily, as many as 40% of elderly patients with mitral valve disease have a history of rheumatic fever or chorea. Other disorders that can cause mitral valve defects include papillary muscle dysfunction secondary to ischemic damage to the heart, calcification of the mitral annulus, and myxomatous degeneration of the mitral valve. Rheumatoid arthritis is a reasonably common condition in the elderly, but mitral valve dysfunction is an uncommon complication even in highly expressed disease.

8. The answer is E. The systolic ejection murmur and delayed carotid upstroke suggest that this patient has aortic stenosis. Vasodilator therapy (e.g., with captopril) in such a patient would decrease total peripheral resistance without necessarily increasing cardiac output, resulting in a severe decrease in blood pressure. Thus, vasodilator therapy would not be indicated until an adequate workup ruled out aortic stenosis as a possible cause of the patient's congestive heart failure. On the other hand, diuretic therapy and digitalization (e.g., with digoxin) should be useful in reducing the patient's congestive symptoms. Definitive surgery or balloon dilatation should be considered once the patient's heart failure has improved.

9. The answer is B. The decision to treat patients (especially the elderly) with antiarrhythmic drugs must be made carefully, in light of the fact that these agents have a limited ability to prevent sudden death and carry a considerable risk of toxicity. However, the high mortality rates associated with certain cardiac arrhythmias justify the risks of this treatment. Up to 30% of patients who survive primary ventricular fibrillation and up to 40% of patients with recurrent sustained ventricular tachycardia die from sudden cardiac death. The mortality rate associated with *torsades de pointes* ventricular tachycardia also is quite high; particular care must be taken when treating elderly patients with this disorder, which most often is due to medications with quinidine-like effects or electrolyte disturbances (e.g., hypokalemia, hypomagnesemia). Patients with an ejection fraction less than 40% and ventricular electrical instability (e.g., complex ventricular ectopy) also are at a high risk for sudden death. Patients with frequent ventricular premature beats and occasional couplets do not necessarily have a poor prognosis; therefore, the risks of antiarrhythmic therapy (including possible exacerbation of the ventricular ectopy) outweigh the benefits of treatment in this situation.

10. The answer is E. The initial evaluation of any patient with hypertension of any type includes a careful medical history and physical examination as well as basic laboratory studies. Measurement of BUN and serum creatinine and urinalysis aid in the evaluation of renal status. In addition, the serum potassium level should be checked to rule out mineralocorticoid-induced hypertension and to provide a baseline value should diuretic therapy be indicated. Because isolated systolic hypertension has been associated with diabetes mellitus and thiazide treatment may worsen hyperglycemia, the serum glucose level also should be checked. Electrocardiography and echocardiography are optional procedures to be carried out if clinical suspicion warrants.

11. The answer is C. All of the vasodilating agents listed in the question are used to treat patients with congestive heart failure—either in combination with or in place of diuretics and digoxin. Nitroglycerin is a direct-acting venodilator that relaxes venous smooth muscle and, thus, reduces preload. Hydralazine is a direct-acting arterial dilator that increases cardiac output by decreasing afterload. Prazosin, captopril, and nifedipine act on both venous and arterial beds and are termed "balanced" vasodilators; prazosin blocks α-adrenergic receptors, captopril inhibits ACE-induced vasoconstriction, and nifedipine is a calcium channel blocker that has marked vasodilatory effects.

12. The answer is B. The cardiovascular response to exercise in a healthy elderly person is different from the response in a younger person. Although it is not certain what factors lead to an age-associated decrease in exercise ability, it is not due to a diminished ability to augment cardiac output. A high level of cardiac output can be achieved in a healthy elderly person; however, the mechanisms used to maintain cardiac output differ dramatically from those used in younger persons. To achieve the same high output, older persons increase heart rate to a lesser extent but increase stroke volume to a greater extent than younger persons. The enhanced stroke volume in older persons is attributed to an increase in end-diastolic volume (to as high as 30% above resting). Because end-systolic volume does not decline greatly in elderly persons, the increased stroke volume is caused by the Frank-Starling mechanism. Ejection fraction increases in younger hearts by reduction in end-systolic volume, which is a more effective mechanism than the reliance on Frank-Starling compensatory effects.

13. The answer is C. Sick sinus syndrome is a disorder of SA node function often associated with varying degrees of sinus exit block, sinus pauses, or even sinus arrest. Patients exhibit severe sinus bradycardia alone or alternating with episodes of supraventricular tachycardia. Electric pacing is the treatment of choice for symptomatic bradycardia; if asymptomatic, a pacemaker still may be considered but is not mandatory. In the symptomatic patient who also has tachycardia, both pacemaker and drug therapy are indicated. However, digoxin alone may further prolong a sinus pause, potentially causing ischemic symptoms. Quinidine should not be used as initial therapy in atrial fibrillation due to the possibility of changing the AV node conduction from 2:1 to 1:1 at a rate greater than 200 beats/min. If pacemaker insertion is indicated, the simplest (i.e., the ventricular demand, or VVI, mode) is adequate for most patients.

14. The answer is D. The postphlebitic syndrome generally presents as a lower leg complication due to a permanent obstruction of the deep venous system. It occurs in 10% of patients with deep venous thrombosis. Physical findings include chronic venous insufficiency, venous valvular incompetence, leg edema, pain, nocturnal cramping, venous claudication, abnormal skin pigmentation, and dermatitis. Stasis ulceration may occur years after the episode of deep venous thrombosis, but it can result in severe progressive disability. Pulmonary embolism is not likely to occur as part of this syndrome, although it can occur after any episode of deep venous thrombosis.

15–18. The answers are: 15-T, 16-F, 17-T, 18-F. Calcification of a congenitally bicuspid aortic valve most commonly results in clinically significant aortic stenosis in the fifth and sixth decades. Calcification of an apparently normal aortic valve most commonly presents as hemodynamically significant aortic stenosis in the seventh and eighth decades. The importance of recognizing the subtle physical signs and clinical manifestations of severe aortic stenosis is underscored by the fact that this defect usually can be cured with aortic valve replacement, even in very old patients. A delayed carotid upstroke is the most reliable sign of severe aortic stenosis. The ejection murmur in severe aortic stenosis usually is harsh and peaks late in systole, when outflow from the left ventricle is at a maximum. However, the murmur may be quite soft, as decreased outflow in the later stages of the disease reduces the intensity of the murmur. The aortic component of S_2 usually is soft or absent due to limited motion of the valve. A diastolic rumble is a finding in mitral stenosis.

19–22. The answers are: 19-F, 20-T, 21-F, 22-T. The mortality rates associated with myocardial infarction are increased greatly—in fact, about doubled—in patients older than 70 years as compared to younger patients. The reasons for this are unclear but seem to represent a combination of factors—some age-related and others not. Elderly patients usually have a more severe presentation, with heart failure, pulmonary edema, and cardiogenic shock. Cardiac rupture also is far more likely in elderly patients, possibly because of an increased prevalence of hypertension, a greater severity of disease, or an age-related change in the usual inflammatory response to infarction. It is not yet certain whether age-related changes in the conduction system affect the likelihood of heart block development after a myocardial infarction; however, the incidence of serious ventricular arrhythmias is not age-related.

23–26. The answers are: 23-F, 24-T, 25-T, 26-F. The calcium channel blocking agents (verapamil, nifedipine, diltiazem) are vasodilators that can be used to enhance or substitute for β blockers in the treatment of angina. Calcium channel blockers act by dilating peripheral veins and arteries, thus decreasing preload and afterload, and by dilating coronary arteries, thus preventing coronary vasospasm. Nifedipine has the greatest peripheral dilating effect and is useful for treating hypertension. Verapamil slows AV node conduction and depresses the rate of the SA node pacemaker, thus making it useful for treating supraventricular tachycardias; it must be used with caution, however, in patients with sick sinus syndrome. Although verapamil is contraindicated in patients with congestive heart failure because it decreases cardiac output, nifedipine and diltiazem can be used safely. In fact, nifedipine actually may enhance cardiac output due to its reduction of afterload.

27–30. The answers are: 27-T, 28-T, 29-T, 30-F. The origin of deep venous thrombosis most often is in the lower extremity venous system. The classic clinical picture includes calf or thigh pain, edema, tenderness, and a positive Homans' sign; however, 50% of patients with proven venous thrombosis have no physical findings in the extremities. Although venography is the most accurate diagnostic technique, Doppler ultrasonography and impedance plethysmography also are highly accurate, provided that the thrombosis occurs above the knee. The treatment of choice for uncomplicated deep venous thrombosis is continuous heparin infusion for 7–10 days, followed by administration of warfarin or subcutaneous administration of heparin for 3–6 months. Radiolabeled fibrinogen scanning is most useful for detecting thrombi in calf veins, but recent calf hematomas, surgical trauma, or inflammatory conditions can give false-positive results. Thrombi in the calf rarely embolize to the lung but occasionally can extend proximally and then embolize. Lower extremity venography can produce negative results in as many as one-third of patients with documented pulmonary embolism.

31–34. The answers are: 31-T, 32-F, 33-T, 34-F. Multifocal atrial tachycardia presents as an irregular supraventricular rhythm with a heart rate between 100 and 200 beats/min. Each QRS complex is preceded by a P wave, but the P wave configuration and PR interval vary from beat to beat. AV block can be present, but the rhythm is not affected by carotid sinus massage. Multifocal atrial tachycardia is a typical rhythm disturbance seen in elderly patients with respiratory failure or multiorgan failure. It is not typically associated with digitalis intoxication but in rare instances can present in this way. Most often, multifocal atrial tachycardia responds to improvement in the general condition of the patient, especially a patient with respiratory failure. If hemodynamic compromise is present, intravenous verapamil is the best available agent; it reduces both atrial and ventricular rates and may convert the arrhythmia to a normal sinus rhythm.

35–38. The answers are: 35-T, 36-F, 37-T, 38-F. Several factors must be considered in the initial management of this elderly man. Appropriate beginning therapy would be to transport him, with intravenous access and monitoring, to the hospital. Although this patient has symptoms that are suggestive of pulmonary edema, he is tolerating the condition with relatively stable vital signs, so immediate synchronized electric cardioversion is not indicated. This treatment may be used later, however, if the patient's symptoms worsen or if it seems an appropriate alternative to the usual drugs that affect AV node conduction to control ventricular rate. Digoxin, verapamil, and propranolol are agents that can inhibit AV node conduction and reduce the ventricular response to atrial fibrillation, allowing the rhythm to self-terminate, which it often does. Verapamil and propranolol should be avoided in this patient, since these agents might further compromise cardiac output. Arterial blood gas analysis is appropriate for assessing this patient's oxygenation and serves as a diagnostic aid in the evaluation of possible causes of the atrial fibrillation (e.g., pulmonary embolism). Anticoagulation is unnecessary when atrial fibrillation has been present for such a short time (i.e., less than 48 hours).

39–42. The answers are: 39-T, 40-T, 41-T, 42-F. Several disease processes can result in atrial fibrillation. Myocardial infarction must be ruled out as it can produce a variety of arrhythmias. Isoenzyme studies can determine with high probability whether a myocardial infarction has occurred. Thyroid hormone excess is a common cause of arrhythmias in the elderly, so thyrotoxicosis also must be ruled out. Echocardiography can identify myocardial abnormalities (e.g., amyloidosis), valvular dysfunction (e.g., mitral or tricuspid stenosis or regurgitation), or obstructing lesions (i.e., atrial myxomas) that may be responsible for new atrial arrhythmias. Although pulmonary embolism may be a causal factor, pulmonary angiography usually is not the first step in making this diagnosis. Arterial blood gas analysis and ventilation and perfusion scanning usually would be performed first if clinical suspicion of pulmonary embolism were present.

43–46. The answers are: 43-T, 44-T, 45-T, 46-T. Some cardiologists believe cardioversion to be the treatment of choice in patients with atrial fibrillation of short duration and in those who do not have significant atrial enlargement or valvular disease. Cardioversion also should be considered in a patient who is not tolerating an arrhythmia. Anticoagulation prior to cardioversion is appropriate if the patient has mitral valve disease, atrial enlargement, an atrial or a ventricular mural thrombus, or a history of thromboembolism. Anticoagulation also should be considered if the atrial fibrillation has been present for longer than 2 days or exists in the setting of cardiomyopathy or thyrotoxicosis. Atrial flutter usually requires less than 100 watt-sec to convert, whereas atrial fibrillation often requires 100–400 watt-sec.

47–50. The answers are: 47-T, 48-T, 49-T, 50-T. The initial consideration of the cause of severe and sudden abdominal pain should include several different organ systems and a host of life-threatening processes. The differential diagnosis is aided in this case by the age of the patient. Atherosclerosis is a common problem in the elderly population and can present as several disorders.

Intestinal angina refers to the acute episodes of mesenteric insufficiency that most commonly result from atherosclerosis of the splanchnic arteries. The pain is analogous to that arising in the myocardium, with angina pectoris, or in the calf muscles, with intermittent claudication; most frequently, the symptoms occur after eating.

Abdominal aortic aneurysm is a very unlikely diagnosis in a person who is younger than 50 years, but it must be considered in older patients due to its lethal nature; up to 80% of symptomatic patients die within 1 year. Acute abdominal pain often develops with a dissecting aneurysm.

Myocardial infarction can be another manifestation of atherosclerosis. Atypical presentation is not unusual in an elderly patient; in particular, inferior myocardial infarction can present solely as abdominal pain due to diaphragmatic irritation.

A perforated viscus also must be considered in a patient with a history of severe abdominal pain.

51–54. The answers are: 51-T, 52-T, 53-T, 54-F. In choosing among diagnostic procedures to be employed in this case, it is important to consider the quality of information that is desired as well as the speed, availability, safety, and cost of the test.

Plain x-rays are safe, inexpensive, and reasonable in the initial evaluation of abdominal pain. These films can be diagnostic of abdominal aneurysm, if characteristic eggshell calcification outlines a mass.

The use of ultrasonography and CT scanning has increased in many diagnostic situations as the quality of the equipment has improved and the cost of the tests has decreased. Both procedures are noninvasive, although contrast medium may be required for CT scanning. Ultrasonography and CT scanning can provide accurate information about the existence, size, and extent of an abdominal aortic aneurysm.

Although aortography has been the diagnostic standard in the past, it is not used as often as a first-line test when ultrasonography and CT scanning are available. Furthermore, when a laminated thrombus is present in the lumen of the aneurysm, aortography may give misleading information as to the size of the deformity.

55–58. The answers are: 55-T, 56-T, 57-T, 58-T. Generally, it is believed that abdominal pain due to an aortic aneurysm is an indication that the lesion is enlarging rapidly and may soon rupture, if rupture has not occurred already. Rupture of an abdominal aortic aneurysm almost inevitably is fatal, thus surgical intervention is mandatory. The operative mortality rate in these situations, however, also is very high (up to 80%); in comparison, elective resection has a mortality rate of less than 5% in most cases. The natural history of aneurysms that exceed 6 cm is a 50% likelihood of rupture over the following 1–2 years. In the elderly patient, the decision to perform elective surgery must take into account the overall health of the patient, as postoperative mortality in the elective setting usually is associated with hypertension, myocardial infarction, or renal failure. In patients over the age of 75 with aneurysms less than 6 cm, an appropriate conservative approach may be to treat the other conditions (especially hypertension) and to follow with regular ultrasonography, proceeding to surgery if the aneurysm enlarges.

5 Hematologic Disorders and Oncologic Diseases

QUESTIONS

Directions: Each question below contains five suggested answers. Choose the **one best** response to each question.

1. In a patient with primary non–oat cell carcinoma of the lung, all of the following factors would preclude surgical treatment EXCEPT

(A) unstable angina
(B) pleural effusion
(C) evidence of significant pulmonary hypertension
(D) vocal cord paralysis
(E) metastases to the ipsilateral hilar lymph nodes

2. The National Conference on Antithrombotic Therapy has identified several characteristics of bleeding that occurs during anticoagulant therapy with warfarin. All of the following statements concerning risks of bleeding during anticoagulant therapy are true EXCEPT

(A) the risk of bleeding is especially high in patients with venous thrombosis
(B) the risk of bleeding is markedly decreased with a less intense anticoagulation regimen
(C) adding dipyridamole to warfarin does not demonstrably increase the risk of bleeding
(D) patients with cerebrovascular disease are most likely to have gastrointestinal bleeding complications
(E) symptomatic bleeding frequently occurs when the PT is in the therapeutic range

3. All of the following statements concerning gastric carcinoma are true EXCEPT

(A) the incidence in the United States has continued to increase over the past 60 years
(B) the incidence is increased in persons with blood group A
(C) atrophic gastritis and gastric polyps are considered premalignant lesions
(D) family members of patients with gastric carcinoma have an increased risk
(E) gross gastrointestinal bleeding is rare

4. Which of the following groups of patients is at highest risk for proximal deep venous thrombosis of the lower extremity?

(A) Patients who recently have undergone total hip replacement
(B) Patients who recently have undergone a neurosurgical procedure
(C) Patients with carcinoma of the lung
(D) Patients with congestive heart failure who are confined to bed
(E) Patients with documented calf vein thrombosis

5. All of the following are risk factors for colorectal carcinoma EXCEPT

(A) age over 50 years
(B) ulcerative colitis
(C) Peutz-Jeghers syndrome
(D) tobacco use
(E) high-calorie, high-fat diet

6. An 82-year-old man whose only significant medical history is a Billroth II procedure for peptic ulcer disease is found to have iron deficiency anemia. The only drug he is taking is aspirin, at a dosage of 6–8 tablets daily for osteoarthritis. Stool examination is negative for occult blood. What is the best initial step in the management of this patient?

(A) Discontinue aspirin and treat with oral iron
(B) Treat with antacids and oral iron
(C) Treat with intramuscular iron
(D) Investigate for iron malabsorption
(E) Investigate the bowel for a bleeding source

7. A 65-year-old man who is scheduled for elective surgery is found to have a hematocrit of 67% and an elevated red cell mass when measured isotopically. Additional studies that would be appropriate in this case include all of the following procedures EXCEPT

(A) arterial blood gas analysis for oxygen saturation
(B) hemoglobin electrophoresis
(C) measurement of serum vitamin B_{12} level
(D) platelet count
(E) liver and spleen scanning

8. All of the following conditions are likely to cause absolute erythrocytosis in elderly persons EXCEPT

(A) high oxygen-affinity hemoglobin
(B) smoker's polycythemia
(C) renal carcinoma
(D) lung carcinoma
(E) severe pulmonary disease

9. Bladder carcinoma in the United States has all of the following characteristics EXCEPT

(A) a higher incidence in men than in women
(B) an association with occupational carcinogens
(C) a squamous cell origin in 90% of cases
(D) a classic presentation of painless hematuria
(E) a high rate of recurrence

10. All of the following statements characterize the acquired sideroblastic anemia that is seen in elderly patients EXCEPT

(A) two populations of erythrocytes typically are seen on peripheral blood smear
(B) treatment with high-dose pyridoxine usually is successful
(C) in 10% of cases the anemia transforms into acute leukemia
(D) drugs and inflammatory diseases are common causes
(E) platelet and leukocyte counts usually are normal

11. Which of the following statements concerning breast cancer is true?

(A) The rate of early detection is highest in women over age 60
(B) Age alone is not a sufficient basis for high-risk screening
(C) Needle biopsy provides a rapid assay of estrogen receptor status
(D) Estrogen receptor status does not affect the relapse rate following mastectomy
(E) Postmenopausal women who do not respond to initial treatment with tamoxifen should receive progesterone or diethylstilbestrol

12. In the elderly, hemolytic anemia most often is the result of an autoimmune process or an adverse drug effect. Which of the following statements best describes autoimmune hemolysis in the elderly?

(A) Cold agglutinin disease is a rare type of autoimmune hemolysis in the elderly
(B) Autoimmune hemolysis is associated with renal cell carcinoma
(C) The direct Coombs' test reliably shows clinical hemolysis to be immune mediated
(D) In most patients with autoimmune syndromes, the hemolysis is predominantly intravascular
(E) Many drug-related causes of hemolysis are indistinguishable clinically from autoimmune hemolysis

13. The incidence of non-Hodgkin's lymphoma rises precipitously after age 40 and is quite high in the elderly. All of the following statements regarding non-Hodgkin's lymphoma are true EXCEPT

(A) painless adenopathy is the most common clinical presentation
(B) previous chemotherapy with alkylating agents increases the risk for tumor development
(C) cytogenetic abnormalities (chromosomal trisomies, deletions, or translocations) are less common in non-Hodgkin's lymphoma than in Hodgkin's disease
(D) most patients have multicentric disease at presentation
(E) the presence of systemic signs is not useful in staging and prognosis

14. Which of the following factors can cause petechiae or purpura in an elderly person without affecting platelet function?

(A) Corticosteroids
(B) Chronic myelogenous leukemia
(C) Carbenicillin
(D) Uremia
(E) Waldenström's macroglobulinemia

15. Which of the following factors in the initial history and physical examination of an elderly patient with macrocytic anemia would best distinguish between folate deficiency and vitamin B_{12} deficiency as the cause of the anemia?

(A) A history of alcoholism
(B) A history of depression
(C) Hypersegmental polymorphonuclear leukocytes on peripheral smear
(D) Peripheral neuropathy and dorsal column disease
(E) Small bowel disorder (e.g., Crohn's disease)

16. Complications of multiple myeloma include all of the following EXCEPT

(A) osteoblastic lesions
(B) renal failure
(C) hypercalcemia
(D) infections
(E) amyloidosis

17. Causes of reactive thrombocytosis include all of the following EXCEPT

(A) iron deficiency
(B) polycythemia vera
(C) splenectomy
(D) rheumatoid arthritis
(E) lung carcinoma

Directions: The groups of questions below consist of an introductory premise or case data followed by four statements that pertain to the information given. Indicate whether each statement is **true** or **false**.

Questions 18–21

The following guidelines for anticoagulation with warfarin have been established by the National Conference on Antithrombotic Therapy.

18. Moderate-dose anticoagulation (PT prolonged to 1.2–1.5 times control) is recommended for prevention of deep venous thrombosis prior to total hip replacement

19. High-dose anticoagulation (PT prolonged to 1.5–2.5 times control) is recommended for treatment of documented proximal deep venous thrombosis in the lower extremity

20. Moderate-dose anticoagulation is recommended for prevention of systemic embolism in the setting of valvular heart disease or prosthetic heart valves

21. Long-term, moderate-dose anticoagulation is now recommended for survivors of acute myocardial infarction to prevent reinfarction

Questions 22–25

Also established by the National Conference on Antithrombotic Therapy are the following guidelines for the use of antiplatelet agents.

22. Aspirin (1 g/day) plus dipyridamole (225 mg/day) is appropriate therapy for preserving graft patency after saphenous vein aortocoronary bypass surgery

23. Aspirin (1 g/day) plus dipyridamole (225 mg/day) is appropriate for prevention of recurrent stroke in patients with completed thrombotic stroke

24. Dipyridamole (up to 400 mg/day) is appropriate for prevention of recurrent systemic embolism in patients with prosthetic heart valves who are not treated successfully with warfarin alone

25. Aspirin (325 mg/day) is appropriate for prevention of myocardial infarction in patients with unstable angina

Questions 26–29

Periodically, adenocarcinoma is discovered in patients in whom the primary origin of the cancer is not known. In such patients, it is important to rule out the following tumors, which are somewhat responsive to therapy.

26. Prostatic carcinoma
27. Breast carcinoma
28. Renal cell carcinoma
29. Adenocarcinoma of the lung

Questions 30–33

The following tests typically are useful for distinguishing anemia of chronic disease from iron deficiency anemia.

30. Serum iron and transferrin levels
31. Serum ferritin level
32. Bone marrow examination
33. Reticulocyte count

Questions 34–37

Carcinoembryonic antigen (CEA) levels are useful in the management of colonic cancers. The following are appropriate uses for CEA in oncologic practice.

34. As a screening test, to distinguish a benign from a malignant colonic lesion
35. As a screening test, to follow families with polyposis syndromes for the appearance of colonic malignancies
36. Preoperatively, to gauge resectability of a colonic neoplasm
37. Postoperatively, as an early indicator of recurrence after resection of a colonic adenocarcinoma

Questions 38–41

A 70-year-old healthy man is found to have a hard, nontender nodule in the prostatic midline on rectal examination. Needle biopsy confirms prostatic adenocarcinoma. Serum acid phosphatase level is normal, pelvic CT scanning is negative for nodal metastases, and radiolabeled bone scanning does not reveal distant metastases. The following are appropriate treatment choices for this patient.

38. Radical prostatectomy
39. Pelvic lymph node biopsy
40. Hormone therapy
41. Radiation therapy

Questions 42–45

The following statements characterize the pathogenesis and clinical course of chronic lymphocytic leukemia.

42. Anemia and thrombocytopenia that occur early in the disease are more likely due to autoimmune factors than to marrow replacement
43. The disease usually is caused by a monoclonal proliferation of T cells
44. Prior exposure to ionizing radiation or alkylating agents is a risk factor for disease development
45. The extent of marrow infiltration by lymphoid elements determines the clinical course

Questions 46–49

Hodgkin's disease in geriatric patients differs from that in younger patients in the following ways.

46. Asymptomatic mediastinal adenopathy is a more common disease presentation
47. Response to combination chemotherapy is less likely to induce a complete remission
48. Drug dosages in combination chemotherapy must be reduced because of decreased bone marrow reserve
49. The disease is more likely to involve extranodal sites

Questions 50–53

The following statements describe factors that contribute to the development of macrocytic anemias.

50. Liver disease can produce macrocytic anemia in the absence of folate or vitamin B_{12} deficiency

51. Chemotherapy can induce macrocytosis

52. Alcohol impairs vitamin B_{12} absorption more than folate absorption

53. Strict vegans (people who eat no meat protein) are more likely to suffer from folate deficiency than from vitamin B_{12} deficiency

ANSWERS AND EXPLANATIONS

1. The answer is E. Surgery is the primary therapy for non–oat cell carcinoma of the lung. The initial and most important concern in treating a patient with this cancer is to determine whether the patient is a candidate for surgery based on the extent of the tumor (resectability) and the medical status of the patient (operability). Accepted criteria for nonresectability include such local contraindications as invasion of the mediastinum (e.g., recurrent laryngeal nerve involvement with vocal cord paralysis, metastases to the mediastinal and contralateral hilar lymph nodes), invasion of the chest wall or pleural involvement (e.g., effusions), and local growth that precludes an adequate surgical margin (e.g., growth within 2 cm of the carina). Metastases to the ipsilateral hilar lymph nodes, however, do not preclude surgery. Patients considered to be at serious operative risk include those with such cardiovascular complications as left ventricular failure, unstable angina, recent myocardial infarction, or ventricular arrhythmia that is unresponsive to drug treatment. Pulmonary contraindications to lung resection include severe obstructive or restrictive lung disease, especially if severe enough to cause pulmonary hypertension. If medical status allows, lung resection should be considered even for very old patients.

2. The answer is D. In the 1986 National Conference on Antithrombotic Therapy (a joint meeting of the American College of Chest Physicians and the National Heart, Lung, and Blood Institute), several risk factors for bleeding complications of long-term anticoagulant therapy were identified. The patient groups found to be at highest risk for anticoagulation-associated bleeding are those with ischemic cerebrovascular or cardiovascular disease and patients with venous thrombosis, probably due to associated risk factors (e.g., hypertension in the former group; cancer, recent surgery, or paraplegia in the latter group). In patients with cerebrovascular disease, the most common site of anticoagulation-associated bleeding is the brain, not the gastrointestinal tract. Clinical bleeding has been shown to occur often in patients when the PT is in the presumed therapeutic range; however, the risk of bleeding is reduced significantly with a lower intensity regimen of anticoagulation (i.e., PT prolonged to 1.2–1.5 times control). The risk of bleeding is not increased significantly by the addition of dipyridamole to warfarin in the treatment of patients with prosthetic heart valve–associated systemic emboli.

3. The answer is A. The incidence of gastric carcinoma in the United States has decreased over the past 60 years, although it remains high in eastern Europe and Japan. The etiology is unknown, but several premalignant conditions have been identified, and a genetic factor is implied by the increased incidence in family members. The incidence of gastric carcinoma also is increased in persons with blood group A and is somewhat decreased in those with blood group O. Anemia from chronic low-grade blood loss is common, but gross gastrointestinal blood loss occurs in only 10% of patients. The prognosis is poor, with only 12% of patients surviving for 5 years.

4. The answer is A. Proximal deep venous thrombosis of the lower extremity occurs in about 40%–70% of patients who recently have undergone total hip replacement. Other patient groups at similar risk for either thigh or calf thrombosis are those undergoing total knee replacement and those with recent hip fractures. Appropriate measures for prevention of deep venous thrombosis in these high-risk groups might include adjusted-dose heparin (to prolong the PTT to the upper end of the therapeutic range), moderate-dose warfarin, and intermittent pneumatic compression. Patients with carcinoma of the lung are at an increased risk for proximal deep venous thrombosis, but the risk does not approach that in the other groups mentioned. As many as 15%–20% of patients with congestive heart failure who are at bed rest and patients who recently have undergone neurosurgical procedures suffer calf vein thrombosis; much less commonly do these groups suffer thigh clots. Pneumatic compression and low-dose subcutaneous heparin are appropriate preventive measures in these patients. Isolated calf vein thrombosis uncommonly extends to proximal veins or causes pulmonary embolism. These thrombi often can be managed without anticoagulation if repeat impedance plethysmography is used to document the lack of proximal extension.

5. The answer is D. Prominent risk factors associated with colorectal carcinoma include advancing age (the incidence begins to rise between the ages of 40 and 50 years and then increases sharply thereafter), inflammatory bowel disease (ulcerative colitis more often than Crohn's disease), and a history of colonic adenoma or cancer of the colon, breast, or female genitalia. Low-fiber, high-calorie, high-fat, and high–meat protein diets also appear to be important contributing factors in the development of colorectal cancers. A higher rate of large bowel cancer also occurs in association with familial syndromes—both the polyposis type (e.g., Gardner's syndrome, familial polyposis, Peutz-Jegher's syndrome) and the nonpolyposis type (e.g., "family cancer syndrome"). Tobacco is not known to predispose to colorectal cancers.

6. The answer is E. In any elderly patient with iron deficiency anemia, a bleeding source must be assumed to be the cause until all potential sources of bleeding have been investigated. Inability to detect blood in the stool does not rule out gastrointestinal blood loss, since it may take years for an occult cecal carcinoma to cause iron deficiency anemia. Another common cause of occult gastrointestinal bleeding—erosive gastritis from treatment with a nonsteroidal anti-inflammatory drug—should be sought in this patient if a lower bowel malignancy is not found. Gastric resection, especially Billroth II anastomosis, can lead to iron deficiency anemia because dietary iron rapidly bypasses the duodenal site where iron is most effectively absorbed; however, such a cause should not be assumed or treated until a bleeding lesion has been excluded.

7. The answer is B. The elevated hematocrit and isotopically confirmed elevated red cell mass in this patient indicate the presence of absolute erythrocytosis. Differential diagnosis requires testing for polycythemia vera, which by convention includes demonstration of a normal arterial oxygen saturation, splenomegaly, an elevated vitamin B_{12} level, elevated platelet and leukocyte levels, and an elevated leukocyte alkaline phosphatase level. Plotting an oxyhemoglobin–dissociation curve is necessary when a patient's erythrocytosis is believed to be due to high oxygen-affinity hemoglobin; hemoglobin electrophoresis, however, does not distinguish these abnormal types of hemoglobin from normal hemoglobin.

8. The answer is D. Lung carcinoma is not a tumor that typically is associated with absolute erythrocytosis, but renal, adrenal, and hepatocellular cancers do cause absolute erythrocytosis via autonomous production of erythropoietin. Hemoglobin variants with increased oxygen affinity do not release oxygen appropriately to tissues, and patients with these variants have compensatory increases in erythropoietin. Some heavy smokers, particularly those who inhale cigar smoke, are found to have high levels of carboxyhemoglobin from inhaled carbon monoxide. Chronic mild elevations in carboxyhemoglobin also are associated with compensatory release of erythropoietin due to poor oxygen release to tissues. Severe pulmonary disease with associated hypoxemia also causes an appropriate increase in erythropoietin release and consequent erythrocytosis.

9. The answer is C. Bladder cancer occurs two to three times more commonly in men than in women and is associated with cigarette smoking and exposure to certain occupational carcinogens (e.g., those found in the rubber, dye, and printing industries). Patients with bladder tumors classically present with painless hematuria, although other symptoms such as bladder infection and irritability may be seen in about 25% of patients. Transitional cell cancer is the main pathologic type found in the United States. In the Middle East, schistosomiasis results in a unique squamous cell bladder cancer, but this is rare in the United States. The tumor sometimes can be managed in the early stages by local removal. However, bladder cancers tend to recur and, therefore, require aggressive follow-up with IVP and cystoscopy.

10. The answer is B. Acquired sideroblastic anemia is an idiopathic disease of older adults. Usually, two erythrocyte populations are found: one normocytic, normochromic and the other macrocytic, hypochromic and basophilic-stippled. Common causes of sideroblastic anemia in the elderly include chronic inflammatory diseases, neoplasia, and drugs that interfere with porphyrin biosynthesis (e.g., alcohol, isoniazid). This disorder develops into acute leukemia in 10% of patients; the only clear-cut risk factor for this transformation is previous chemotherapy with an alkylating agent. Pyridoxine in large dosages occasionally is successful therapy for the hereditary variety but rarely is helpful in acquired sideroblastic anemia. Platelet and leukocyte counts typically are normal in this disease.

11. The answer is A. The incidence of breast cancer increases steadily with age. If for no other reason, elderly women qualify as a high-risk group that should be screened for breast cancer. However, elderly women tend to have a better prognosis than younger women, should breast cancer develop, since lesions often are detected early. With regular mammography (every 1 or 2 years), annual breast examination, and monthly self-examination, there is a higher rate of detection of minimal cancers and, thus, a better chance of cure. An advantage of mammography in elderly women is its increased ability to detect lumps against the low-density background of predominantly fatty breast tissue in older women. The diagnosis of breast cancer is made by biopsy—preferably excisional biopsy. Needle biopsy is useful only when a positive diagnosis is made; it does, however, provide a rapid histologic assay of the cancer but does not provide for evaluation of estrogen receptor (ER) status. ER status is an important biologic determinant of tumor response, which has therapeutic and prognostic value; ER-positive tumors generally are associated with a higher survival rate. Generally, patients with positive ER assays have longer relapse-free survival following mastectomy than those with negative assays. Postmenopausal women with advanced disease, especially those older than 60 years with ER-positive tumors, are prime candidates for palliative hormone therapy. The initial treatment of choice is tamoxifen. Women who do not respond to tamoxifen, however, generally do not respond to other forms of hormone therapy and should be given chemotherapy.

12. The answer is E. Many drug-related causes of hemolysis are immune mediated (e.g., penicillin or cephalosporins in hapten-type hemolysis) and are indistinguishable clinically from autoimmune hemolysis. Cold agglutinin disease in the young is associated with mycoplasmal pneumonia or infectious mononucleosis, but this form of hemolysis is uncommon. Cold agglutinin disease is more common in the elderly and may be associated with lymphoproliferative or autoimmune diseases. There is no association with renal cell carcinoma, however. In at least 10% of patients, the direct Coombs' test is negative at the time that significant immune-mediated hemolysis is ongoing. In most cases, hemolysis occurs in the spleen or reticuloendothelial system rather than in the bloodstream.

13. The answer is C. Lymphocyte cytogenetic abnormalities almost always are found in non-Hodgkin's lymphoma if searched for on high-resolution microscopy. No characteristic cytogenetic abnormalities are found in Hodgkin's disease. Painless adenopathy is the most common presentation of both Hodgkin's disease and non-Hodgkin's lymphoma, although the enlarged nodes can produce signs and symptoms in both conditions; compression of adjacent veins by enlarged inguinal nodes can lead to deep venous thrombosis, and enlarged retroperitoneal nodes can lead to abdominal pain and distension. Prior chemotherapy with alkylating agents is a well-known risk factor for the development of non-Hodgkin's lymphoma. Immune functional impairment (e.g., due to hereditary syndromes or AIDS) also is a risk factor, and infectious causes (e.g., Epstein-Barr virus, which causes Burkitt's lymphoma) and familial clustering of cases have been described. Most patients (90%) present with multicentric disease and extranodal sites (e.g., liver, spleen), indicating already advanced disease. Although systemic features (e.g., weight loss, fever, night sweats) are associated with a worse prognosis and affect treatment decisions in Hodgkin's disease, the same is not true in non-Hodgkin's lymphoma.

14. The answer is A. Corticosteroids cause subcutaneous atrophy and accelerate the natural reduction in vascular supportive tissue seen in old age. Thus, they accentuate senile purpura rather than interfere with platelet function. All of the other factors listed cause abnormalities of platelet structure or function, which can lead to hemorrhage. In chronic myelogenous leukemia, abnormal platelets are produced; carbenicillin, penicillin, and other β-lactam drugs can interfere with normal platelet function, as can aspirin and other nonsteroidal anti-inflammatory agents; uremia and dysproteinemia also cause platelet dysfunction.

15. The answer is D. The presence of peripheral neuropathy and dorsal column disease is called "combined systems disease" and is quite suggestive of vitamin B_{12} deficiency. Patients present with numbness and tingling in the lower extremities as well as a broad-based gait; ataxia, weakness, and hyperreflexia appear as the posterolateral spinal cord becomes affected. Atrophic glossitis and a family history of pernicious anemia are other factors in the initial history and physical examination that would make vitamin B_{12} deficiency more likely than folate deficiency. A history of alcholism is more suggestive of folate deficiency, since alcohol impairs folate absorption, but it certainly is not specific. Depression can be seen in either deficiency state, and hypersegmental polymorphonuclear leukocytes are found on peripheral blood smear in any megaloblastic state. Small bowel or ileal disease impairs the absorption of both folate and vitamin B_{12}.

16. The answer is A. Patients with multiple myeloma most frequently present with an abnormal monoclonal protein (M protein), which is detected in the blood, urine, or both. In addition, myeloma cell–induced bone resorption results in weakened bone, osteolytic lesions, and fractures. The M protein exists in high concentrations in the kidney and acts as a nephrotoxin, contributing (along with hyperuricemia, dehydration, and hypercalcemia) to renal failure in many patients. The myeloma cells also secrete an osteoclast-stimulating factor, which causes hypercalcemia due to calcium resorption from bone. Also, myeloma leads to acquired hypogammaglobulinemia, which predisposes patients to infection. Finally, immunocytic amyloidosis (i.e., the infiltration of organs by light chains) occurs in 15% of cases of myeloma, with cardiac or renal involvement being a common cause of death in these patients. Osteoblastic lesions rarely occur in myeloma.

17. The answer is B. In polycythemia vera and other myeloproliferative disorders (e.g., chronic myelogenous leukemia, essential thrombocythemia), increased platelet counts result from autonomous production. The incidence of myeloproliferative disorders rises with age. In these conditions, platelet counts may increase to levels ranging from 1,000,000 to 3,000,000, and the increased number may contribute to an increased potential for vascular thrombosis; in addition, qualitative platelet function defects can lead to bleeding or thrombosis. Conversely, in reactive disorders, increased platelet production results from some stimulus, qualitative platelet function remains normal, and bleeding or thrombosis are unusual even with very high platelet counts. Iron deficiency and splenectomy both are such stimuli, and chronic inflammatory and neoplastic states are well-known causes of reactive thrombocytosis.

18–21. The answers are: 18-T, 19-F, 20-T, 21-F. In the 1986 National Conference on Antithrombotic Therapy (NCAT), guidelines were established for the use of anticoagulation in a variety of clinical settings. Current NCAT recommendations support that the high (40%–70%) risk of deep venous thrombosis in the setting of total hip replacement warrants prophylactic anticoagulation with adjusted-dose heparin (to upper ranges of PTT) or with moderate-dose warfarin (PT prolonged to 1.2–1.5 times control, when the PT reagent is rabbit brain thromboplastin).

Moderate-dose warfarin also is recommended as appropriate therapy for proximal deep venous thrombosis. The lesser degree of PT prolongation offers acceptable prophylaxis against proximal clot extension or pulmonary embolism in venous thrombosis and minimizes bleeding complications. Similarly, moderate-dose anticoagulation with warfarin appears to offer a reduced risk of hemorrhage and provides acceptable prophylaxis against systemic emboli in patients with valvular heart disease or prosthetic heart valves.

Although popular in the past, long-term anticoagulation with warfarin is not recommended for survivors of acute myocardial infarction, either to prevent reinfarction or to prolong life, because evidence of benefit is marginal and risks, cost, and inconvenience are substantial. Antiplatelet treatment (with aspirin 325 mg every other day) may be useful in this setting, in light of the very recent findings that suggest a reduced risk of myocardial infarction in middle-aged physicians so treated.

22–25. The answers are: 22-T, 23-F, 24-T, 25-T. Both aspirin and dipyridamole have been used in most clinical studies assessing saphenous vein patency following coronary artery bypass grafting, and the combination appears to be effective. It is possible that aspirin alone also may be effective, but the combined treatment is more widely accepted in this situation.

Aspirin without dipyridamole is considered to be appropriate, however, for prevention of stroke in patients with transient ischemic attack as well as for prevention of recurrent stroke in patients with prior completed thrombotic cerebrovascular accident.

When dipyridamole is added to warfarin for prophylaxis against recurrent systemic emboli in patients with prosthetic heart valves, trials show a benefit without an increased risk of bleeding. This combination is preferred to aspirin plus warfarin because of the higher risk for gastrointestinal bleeding with the latter regimen.

Finally, aspirin at a dosage of 1 g/day clearly is effective for preventing myocardial infarction in patients with unstable angina, probably by preventing the adherence of platelets to atheromatous plaques.

26–29. The answers are: 26-T, 27-T, 28-F, 29-F. Advanced prostatic carcinoma has a high rate of initial response to hormone manipulation (administration of exogenous estrogens, orchiectomy) and, thus, should be sought in men who have evidence of adenocarcinoma with no known primary origin. Hormone therapy has been shown to be palliative in most patients and to produce tumor regression in almost half of men treated. Likewise, breast carcinoma should be sought in women, as objective response to hormone manipulation is quite high—especially in women who are older than 60 years and have tumors that are positive for estrogen receptors. In those who do not respond to or are not candidates for hormone therapy, chemotherapy or a combination of both treatments may offer effective palliation. Thyroid carcinoma also should be sought in patients with a tumor of unknown primary origin, as it is responsive to systemic therapy in many cases. Despite isolated reports of successful treatment, adenocarcinoma of the lung and renal cell carcinoma remain fairly refractory neoplasms.

30–33. The answers are: 30-F, 31-T, 32-T, 33-F. In an elderly person, it is important to distinguish anemia that is associated with chronic inflammatory disease (e.g., rheumatoid arthritis, serious infection) from iron deficiency anemia, as the latter most frequently results from occult gastrointestinal bleeding. In typical iron deficiency anemia, the serum iron level falls and the serum iron-binding capacity (serum transferrin concentration) increases, leading to a decrease in percentage saturation (serum iron/serum iron-binding capacity = % saturation). In anemia of chronic disease, the serum iron level falls and the serum transferrin level decreases; however, percentage saturation is not sufficiently different from that typically seen in iron deficiency anemia to be a useful discriminator. Serum ferritin levels are believed to reflect levels of storage iron and, hence, are normal or elevated in anemia of chronic disease but low in iron deficiency anemia. This test is unreliable, however, when iron deficiency coexists with anemia of chronic disease. In this situation, the only adequate discriminator is a bone marrow specimen that is stained to identify iron present in macrophages. Reticulocyte counts typically are low in both of these hypoproliferative disorders.

34–37. The answers are: 34-F, 35-F, 36-T, 37-T. Carcinoembryonic antigen (CEA) was discovered first in embryonal gut tissues. In clinical medicine, CEA is a tumor marker that initially was found to be elevated in serum in association with colorectal carcinoma. However, elevated serum CEA levels (i.e., > 5.0 mg/ml) also have been found in association with other malignancies (e.g., gastric carcinoma, breast carcinoma) as well as other conditions (e.g., heavy cigarette smoking, alcoholic liver disease). Thus, CEA is not as useful a marker for colonic carcinoma as initially predicted, although it still has some value. Elevated levels of CEA in the setting of colonic carcinoma imply that the disease has penetrated through the bowel wall. Preoperatively, CEA can be used to predict the outcome of surgery for colorectal carcinoma: If levels are elevated, the prognosis for surgical cure is poor. Postoperatively, CEA can be used to gauge the completeness of tumor resection: If elevated levels do not fall, occult metastases probably are present. CEA levels also are useful for measuring the response of metastatic disease to treatment. Finally, an increased CEA level is the most accurate predictor of recurrence of colorectal disease after resection. CEA levels are not useful for screening families with polyposis syndromes or for distinguishing benign from malignant colonic lesions.

38–41. The answers are: 38-T, 39-T, 40-F, 41-T. The treatment of prostatic carcinoma is tailored to the staging of the tumor. Stage A disease is not palpable but is discovered on routine histopathology after surgery performed for prostatic hyperplasia. Stage B is a palpable nodule on routine rectal examination, stage C reflects extension beyond the prostatic capsule, and stage D implies metastatic disease. Any patient with an elevated serum acid phosphatase level is considered to have stage D disease.

This patient presumably has stage B prostatic carcinoma or early stage C disease. Either radiation therapy or radical prostatectomy would offer a reasonable chance for cure if pelvic nodes are not involved by microscopic metastases (stage D). Many urologists would choose one of these treatments for this patient, whereas others would sample pelvic nodes to look for metastatic disease not evident on CT scanning. Hormone therapy (e.g., exogenous estrogen, orchiectomy, LHRH analogue treatment) is appropriate only for palliative treatment of stage D disease.

42–45. The answers are: 42-T, 43-F, 44-F, 45-T. Chronic lymphocytic leukemia most commonly is a monoclonal neoplasm of mature but dysfunctional B cells that accumulate in the tissues and peripheral blood. The etiology of the disease is unclear, but a genetic predisposition is possible. Exposure to alkylating agent chemotherapy or ionizing radiation does not increase the risk for disease development, as it does for acute and chronic myeloid leukemia.

Chronic lymphocytic leukemia is difficult to stage; disease progression is gauged by the number of involved lymph node areas and the amount of bone marrow infiltration. Anemia and thrombocytopenia generally imply advanced disease due to marrow infiltration, and the extent of such infiltration typically determines the prognosis. However, autoimmune hemolysis, thrombocytopenia, or both, occasionally occur in chronic lymphocytic leukemia, usually early in the course.

Most patients die due to recurrent infections (related to neutropenia or hypogammaglobulinemia), bleeding from thrombocytopenia, or lymphocytic infiltration of vital organs. Patients generally are treated when the disease produces symptoms or causes progressive marrow infiltration. Aggressive treatment (combination chemotherapy) has not been shown to be more effective than conservative therapy (a single alkylating agent or corticosteroids).

46–49. The answers are: 46-F, 47-T, 48-T, 49-T. Hodgkin's disease has a characteristic bimodal age distribution. The first peak in incidence occurs between the ages of 15 and 30 years, and the second peak occurs after age 50 years. In general, Hodgkin's disease has a more aggressive course in older patients than in younger ones.

Asymptomatic mediastinal adenopathy is a more common disease presentation in those younger than 35 years and most often is associated with the nodular sclerosis histopathologic subtype. The nodular sclerosis type usually is confined to nodal sites, in contrast to the mixed cellularity and lymphocyte-depleted histopathologic varieties, which are seen more often in the geriatric age-group and usually involve extranodal sites. Older patients more often present with extensive intra-abdominal involvement, especially of the liver and spleen. Combination chemotherapy is less likely to induce complete remission in elderly patients, because the histopathologic classification in these patients is less favorable and because drug dosages often cannot be given at full, recommended amounts due to the decreased marrow reserves of these patients.

50–53. The answers are: 50-T, 51-T, 52-F, 53-F. Macrocytic anemias are characterized by abnormally large erythrocytes. Three mechanisms are linked to the development of macrocytic anemia: accelerated erythropoiesis (e.g., response to chronic hemolysis), increased membrane surface area, and defective DNA synthesis.

Patients with severe liver disease incorporate abnormal amounts of cholesterol and phospholipids into erythrocyte membranes, leading to a characteristic target-cell appearance of erythrocytes in the peripheral blood. Chemotherapy with antimetabolites (e.g., methotrexate, azathioprine) interferes with DNA synthesis and can lead to macrocytosis. Alcohol interferes directly with folate metabolism, perhaps by blocking the enterohepatic circulation of folate as well as folate release from tissue stores; alcoholism is a common cause of clinical folate deficiency. Alcohol can impair vitamin B_{12} absorption but does not cause a deficiency state in the absence of other predisposing factors. Strict vegans are more likely to suffer vitamin B_{12} deficiency, since meat and dairy products are the best sources of vitamin B_{12}. Green leafy vegetables are rich in folate, so vegans would be unlikely to experience folate deficiency.

6
Neurologic Disorders

QUESTIONS

Directions: Each question below contains five suggested answers. Choose the **one best** response to each question.

1. An 82-year-old man is seen because of the sudden onset of back pain that has persisted for several days. He also complains of ache in his legs. Initial evaluation reveals a temperature of 102° F, hyporeflexia in the lower extremities, and impaired sensation to pinprick along the lateral aspect of the calves and feet. This patient's signs and symptoms are most suggestive of

(A) spinal meningioma
(B) encephalitis
(C) spinal epidural abscess
(D) diskitis
(E) meningitis

2. A 72-year-old diabetic man presents with a 2-week history of double vision and clinical evidence of a third cranial nerve palsy. Which of the following features is most helpful in determining whether the cause is diabetes or an aneurysm requiring surgical evaluation?

(A) Weakness of inward and downward gaze
(B) Weakness of inward and upward gaze
(C) Ptosis
(D) Pupillary size
(E) Retinopathy

3. In a 67-year-old man, a history of bilateral proximal and distal leg pain and weakness with prolonged standing is most suggestive of

(A) lumbar disk-related S1 radiculopathy
(B) lumbar spinal stenosis
(C) peripheral neuropathy
(D) polymyositis
(E) peripheral vascular disease

4. Hypertensive encephalopathy is an acute neurologic complication of severe hypertension. All of the following are common signs and symptoms of hypertensive encephalopathy EXCEPT

(A) acute onset of confusion and delirium
(B) focal or generalized convulsions
(C) papilledema
(D) retinal hemorrhage
(E) flaccid hemiplegia

5. Which of the following statements best characterizes cardioembolic cerebral infarction?

(A) Mitral annulus calcification is an increasingly recognized finding associated with cardioembolic stroke in elderly persons
(B) Cardioembolic stroke typically is preceded by one or more transient ischemic attacks
(C) When hemorrhage follows cardioembolic stroke, CT scanning provides an early diagnosis
(D) Atrial fibrillation rarely causes cardioembolic stroke in the absence of mitral stenosis
(E) Cardioembolic stroke occurs more often in the anterior than in the middle cerebral territory

6. Herpes zoster is relatively common in the elderly. The most common neurologic complication of herpes zoster is

(A) facial paralysis
(B) segmental myelitis
(C) cerebral vasculitis
(D) postherpetic neuralgia
(E) focal encephalitis

7. The most important risk factor for stroke in the elderly is

(A) hypertension
(B) cigarette smoking
(C) hypercholesterolemia
(D) diabetes mellitus
(E) moderate alcohol consumption

8. Giant cell (temporal) arteritis, an inflammatory vasculitis of the cranial artery circulation, is rare before age 50. All of the following statements regarding giant cell arteritis are true EXCEPT

(A) the most frequent presenting symptoms are headache and claudication of the jaw muscles
(B) erythrocyte sedimentation rate is an important screening test
(C) blindness is a frequent complication in untreated cases
(D) definitive diagnosis is provided by temporal arteriography
(E) the treatment of choice is corticosteroids

9. Which of the following statements is true regarding herpes simplex virus-1 (HSV-1) encephalitis?

(A) HSV-1 encephalitis occurs most commonly during the summer months
(B) HSV-1 encephalitis usually occurs in association with active herpes infection elsewhere in the body
(C) Electroencephalography is the most helpful early neurodiagnostic test for HSV-1 encephalitis
(D) Definitive diagnosis of HSV-1 encephalitis is provided by CSF culture
(E) The number of erythrocytes in the CSF aids in discriminating HSV-1 encephalitis from other infections that mimic it

10. The differential diagnosis of normal pressure hydrocephalus includes all of the following disorders EXCEPT

(A) Alzheimer's disease
(B) Parkinson's disease
(C) alcohol-related cerebellar disease
(D) depression
(E) multi-infarct dementia

11. All of the following factors suggest the likelihood of a good shunt outcome for an elderly patient with normal pressure hydrocephalus EXCEPT

(A) an identifiable cause
(B) the presence of dementia and abnormal gait without incontinence
(C) a short duration of symptoms
(D) absence of cerebral atrophy on CT scanning
(E) temporary improvement following lumbar puncture

12. The syndrome of parkinsonism includes all of the following features EXCEPT

(A) pill-rolling tremor
(B) dysmetria
(C) bradykinesia
(D) cogwheel rigidity
(E) festinating gait

13. Shy-Drager syndrome is best defined as a syndrome combining parkinsonism with

(A) progressive supranuclear palsy
(B) severe autonomic insufficiency
(C) dementia
(D) normal pressure hydrocephalus
(E) seizure disorder

14. Amaurosis fugax most frequently is caused by atherosclerotic carotid artery disease. However, an elderly patient who presents with amaurosis fugax should be evaluated for which of the following potential causes of this disorder?

(A) Pseudotumor cerebri
(B) Giant cell arteritis
(C) Retinal detachment
(D) Migraine
(E) Pituitary adenoma

15. All of the following statements regarding Meige's syndrome (facial dystonia) are true EXCEPT

(A) the involuntary movements usually involve the muscles of the eyes, face, and jaw
(B) bright lights aggravate dystonia of the eye muscles
(C) functional blindness can occur in severe cases
(D) surgery usually is successful in relieving the dystonia
(E) benzodiazepine therapy can produce moderate improvement in patients who are not candidates for surgery

16. Common causes of syncope in the elderly include all of the following drugs and disorders EXCEPT

(A) amitryptyline
(B) methyldopa
(C) COPD
(D) diabetes
(E) Shy-Drager syndrome

17. The tremor that is seen most frequently in the elderly is a manifestation of

(A) old age
(B) medication-related side effects
(C) Parkinson's disease
(D) cerebellar disease
(E) hyperthyroidism

18. All of the following statements regarding chronic subdural hematoma are true EXCEPT

(A) the onset of symptoms may be weeks after minor head trauma
(B) headache is the initial symptom in most patients
(C) lateralizing neurologic signs may be late manifestations
(D) angiography is required to exclude this diagnosis
(E) dialysis patients are at increased risk

19. Amyotrophic lateral sclerosis is a progressive degenerative disease of older adults. All of the following statements characterize this disease EXCEPT

(A) the degenerative process is confined to pyramidal motor neurons
(B) both upper and lower motor neurons are affected
(C) a hallmark is fasciculations of the muscles
(D) urinary incontinence is an early manifestation
(E) patients may experience uncontrollable laughing and crying

20. Cervical spondylosis is the most common cause of cervical myelopathy in middle-aged and older persons. The disorder develops insidiously, with all of the following characteristics EXCEPT

(A) symmetrical involvement
(B) fasciculations and areflexia in upper extremities
(C) increased tendon reflexes in lower extremities
(D) sensory loss in both upper and lower extremities
(E) slow, stiff gait

21. All of the following are significant prognostic factors for a patient who has just suffered a stroke EXCEPT

(A) the age of the patient
(B) the presence of underlying cardiovascular disease
(C) the particular artery involved
(D) the degree of consciousness of the patient during the acute phase
(E) the degree of neurologic deficit suffered

Questions 22 and 23

A 60-year-old man complains of weakness and stiffness in his left arm. Also, on rare occasions he has difficulty lifting his left foot. Physical examination reveals some stiffness in limb movement, a slight tremor, and impaired fine finger movement in the left hand. Early Parkinson's disease is suspected.

22. The diagnostic workup should begin with which of the following tests?

(A) Lumbar puncture
(B) X-ray of the cervical spine
(C) Electromyography of the left arm
(D) Doppler ultrasonography of the left arm
(E) None of the above

The patient's history and clinical examination are consistent with mild, unilateral Parkinson's disease. His symptoms are not severe enough to warrant drug treatment, although he is advised by his physician that treatment may be needed later. After 1½ years, the patient returns with prominent tremor as well as poor coordination and cogwheel rigidity in his left arm. Occasionally, his right arm shakes also.

23. What is the best choice of therapy at this time?

(A) Levodopa
(B) Amantadine
(C) Bromocriptine
(D) Trihexyphenidyl
(E) Amantadine plus trihexyphenidyl

Questions 24–26

A 76-year-old diabetic woman complains of left arm pain and numbness that have persisted for 6 weeks. She awakens at night with tingling in the arm and hand accompanied by a dull ache, which she relieves by shaking her hand. She also notes some weakness of her left hand, which occasionally causes her to drop objects. Physical examination reveals soft bilateral carotid bruits, moderate limitation of neck motion, and decreased sensation to pinprick of the palmar side of the first 4 digits of the left hand. Motor strength, including thumb apposition, is normal, there is no apparent thenar atrophy, and reflexes are intact.

24. What is the most appropriate diagnostic test at this time?

(A) Electromyelography and nerve conduction velocity (EMG/NCV) studies
(B) Cervical myelography
(C) Cervical spine x-ray
(D) Hand and wrist x-ray
(E) Noninvasive carotid studies

25. The diagnosis of carpal tunnel syndrome eventually is made. Appropriate treatments to consider include all of the following EXCEPT

(A) local corticosteroid injection
(B) systemic corticosteroids
(C) surgical decompression
(D) nonsteroidal anti-inflammatory medication
(E) wrist splinting

26. Factors that predispose to the development of carpal tunnel syndrome include all of the following disorders EXCEPT

(A) diabetes
(B) hypothyroidism
(C) amyloidosis
(D) rheumatoid arthritis
(E) osteoporosis

Directions: The groups of questions below consist of an introductory premise or case data followed by four statements that pertain to the information given. Indicate whether each statement is **true** or **false**.

Questions 27–30

It is important to attempt to distinguish between transient ischemic attacks (TIAs) of the carotid arteries and TIAs of the vertebrobasilar circulation, as the treatment and prognosis of the two differ. The following statements describe differentiating characteristics of the two types of TIAs.

27. TIAs of the carotid arteries lead to stroke more often than do TIAs of the vertebrobasilar circulation

28. Binocular visual defects and bilateral sensorimotor disturbances are characteristic of vertebrobasilar TIAs but not of carotid TIAs

29. Transient global amnesia is characteristic of carotid TIAs but not of vertebrobasilar TIAs

30. Loss of consciousness is characteristic of both types of TIAs

Questions 31–34

Although idiopathic parkinsonism is most frequent, drug-induced parkinsonism is not uncommon, with antipsychotic agents the major offenders. The following statements describe the parkinsonian state induced by these agents.

31. Antipsychotic agents induce parkinsonism by depleting dopamine stores in the dopaminergic nerve terminals in the striatum

32. The syndrome is most likely to occur within the first month of antipsychotic therapy

33. The syndrome responds readily to levodopa therapy

34. Neurologic effects resolve with discontinuation of antipsychotic agents

Questions 35–38

Progressive supranuclear palsy can be best distinguished from Parkinson's disease on the basis of the following oculomotor findings.

35. Impaired upward gaze

36. Impaired downward gaze

37. Impaired lateral gaze

38. Impaired convergence

Questions 39–42

An 85-year-old man is seen because of episodes of dizziness. During some of these episodes, he has fainted. The medical history reveals no drugs or underlying disorders that might produce orthostatic hypotension or vasodepressor episodes in this patient, and physical examination reveals normal orthostatic vital signs. In an effort to determine the cause of this patient's syncopal episodes, the following procedures should be performed.

39. Serum electrolyte studies

40. CT scanning of the brain

41. Skull x-ray

42. Holter monitoring

Questions 43–46

Weakness is one of the most common symptoms of neuromuscular disease in elderly patients. The following disorders should be considered in the differential diagnosis of muscle weakness.

43. Guillain-Barré syndrome

44. Myasthenia gravis

45. Polymyositis

46. Polymyalgia rheumatica

Questions 47–50

The National Conference on Antithrombotic Therapy has established guidelines for the use of anticoagulants in cerebrovascular disease. According to these guidelines, anticoagulation (not antiplatelet therapy) is indicated for prevention or treatment of stroke in the following settings.

47. A patient who is experiencing transient ischemic attacks of presumed thrombotic origin

48. A patient with a progressing thrombotic stroke

49. A patient with a completed thrombotic stroke

50. A patient with endocarditis of a native heart valve

ANSWERS AND EXPLANATIONS

1. The answer is C. The triad of back pain, fever, and neurologic dysfunction in the lower extremities of this patient strongly suggests lumbar epidural abscess. This uncommon event is an important neurologic emergency; without prompt diagnosis and appropriate therapy, permanent neurologic damage occurs. The outcome usually is good, however, if surgical drainage and spinal cord decompression are performed and appropriate antibiotics are given before paraplegia occurs. Hyporeflexia is characteristic of a cauda equina lesion; hyperreflexia would be expected if the extradural mass pressed on the spinal cord itself. The most common infective agent of spinal epidural abscess is *Staphylococcus aureus*.

The differential diagnosis of spinal epidural abscess includes several disorders. Although meningitis may produce back pain, headache and stiff neck are more common. Diskitis is disk inflammation mainly seen in spondyloarthropathies; although back pain and fever are characteristic, neurologic compression syndromes are not. A spinal meningioma can produce back pain and neurologic dysfunction but would not be expected to produce fever. Encephalitis would not be included in the differential diagnosis; clinical features most commonly include altered consciousness, behavior changes, and seizures.

2. The answer is D. Third cranial nerve palsy is characterized by a variety of functional disturbances of the oculomotor nerve, including dilation of the pupils, ptosis, and weakness of inward gaze (upward and downward). Several disorders may cause third cranial nerve palsy; some of the more common causes include a midbrain lesion, nerve infarction (due to diabetes mellitus or hypertension), and intracranial aneurysm. Distinguishing between diabetes and aneurysm is aided by the presence or absence of pupillary dysfunction. The nerve fibers that control pupillary constriction lie on the outside of the oculomotor nerve, making them more vulnerable to compression (as occurs in aneurysm) and less vulnerable to ischemic insult (as occurs in diabetes). Thus, pupillary size helps distinguish between these two types of insult. Patients with aneurysms rarely have normal-sized pupils when they present with third nerve palsies. However, a few cases have been described in which the pupil was not dilated at the time of initial complaints. After 1 week without pupillary changes, aneurysm is extremely unlikely (this patient came in 2 weeks after first symptoms). Retinopathy does not distinguish between these two causative disorders. Extraocular muscle palsies and ptosis do not distinguish between the two disorders.

3. The answer is B. Lumbar spinal stenosis is a condition seen in elderly adults that is due to extensive overgrowth of bone and disk space narrowing in the lumbar spine. The bone overgrowth and degenerative disk changes narrow the spinal canal and constrict the cauda equina as well as the nerve roots as they exit at the foramina. Although lumbar back pain is a common complaint, this syndrome is suggested most by the worsening of pain upon standing or walking, especially when the pain radiates down both legs and is accompanied by a sensation of increasing fatigue "marching" up the legs with ambulation. Vascular claudication typically is considered to be the cause, since patients must stop walking and wait for the leg pain and fatigue to subside before continuing. However, peripheral leg pulses are abnormal in this condition whereas they are normal in lumbar spinal stenosis. Also, standing upright typically does not worsen vascular claudication but may worsen or cause pain in the spinal stenosis syndrome. This man's symptoms are not consistent with an S1 radiculopathy, as that syndrome is unilateral and associated with sensory loss of the lateral and plantar aspects of the foot, loss of ankle reflex, and loss of plantar flexion. Peripheral neuropathies are predominantly sensory and distal. Motor complaints, when present, are not affected by standing. Polymyositis involves proximal muscle weakness (i.e., difficulty rising from a sitting position) and usually is not accompanied by pain.

4. The answer is E. The use of effective antihypertensive drugs has made hypertensive encephalopathy less common. However, it is a medical emergency that requires prompt lowering of the blood pressure, which usually has a diastolic reading above 125 mm Hg. Hypertensive encephalopathy is recognized clinically as a rapid onset of confusion and delirium often accompanied by focal or generalized convulsions, which may progress to stupor or coma. Examination usually reveals papilledema and retinal hemorrhage. Congestive heart failure and renal insufficiency often accompany the encephalopathy because of end-organ damage by accelerated hypertension. Transient focal neurologic signs, such as hemiparesis and hemianopia, may occur; however, severe and persistent signs, such as flaccid hemiplagia, are not characteristic of hypertensive encephalopathy and should suggest cerebral hemorrhage.

5. The answer is A. Cerebral infarction may occur due to an embolic or thrombotic occlusion of an intracerebral artery. The most common causes of embolic cerebral infarction are cardiac in origin, the most important of which is an endocardial mural thrombus related to myocardial infarction. Atrial fibrillation is another common cardiac cause, which may or may not be associated with mitral stenosis. An increasingly recognized cause of cardioembolic stroke in elderly patients is mitral annulus calcification (a degenerative process that occurs solely in this age-group). Cardioembolic stroke involves the carotid circulation more often than the vertebrobasilar circulation and the middle cerebral territory more often than the anterior territory. It is unusual for this event to be preceded by one or a series of transient ischemic attacks. There is a tendency for spontaneous hemorrhagic transformation of cardioembolic cerebral infarctions; unfortunately, CT scanning usually is not helpful in identifying hemorrhage in the acute phase (i.e., less than 12 hours after the onset of stroke).

6. The answer is D. The incidence of herpes zoster (shingles) increases steadily with age; persons older than 60 years are affected at least twice as often as younger persons. The incidence is drastically increased, however, in persons with depressed immunity (e.g., due to lymphoma or chemotherapy). Neurologic complications of herpes zoster that are most likely to occur in immunocompetent persons include chronic severe pain (referred to as postherpetic neuralgia), facial paralysis (due to an infection of the geniculate ganglion of the facial nerve, also referred to as the Ramsay Hunt syndrome), segmental myelitis, and cerebral vasculitis. Recent evidence suggests that postherpetic neuralgia, a particularly troublesome condition that affects more than 50% of elderly patients, may be reduced by early treatment with acyclovir. Focal encephalitis is an uncommon complication of herpes zoster, occurring primarily in immunocompromised persons.

7. The answer is A. The most powerful risk factor for stroke is completely unavoidable in that it is age itself. By far the most important avoidable risk factor in the elderly, however, is hypertension. Hypertension plays a causative role in almost all types of stroke, with the exception of certain types of embolic stroke. Other important avoidable factors that predispose to stroke in the elderly are heart disease and diabetes. Cigarette smoking and moderate alcohol consumption seem to be additional risk factors; however, it is impossible to evaluate these factors independent of other, more significant ones. The risk of stroke in the elderly population appears to be relatively unaffected by serum cholesterol levels.

8. The answer is D. Giant cell arteritis (also known as temporal arteritis) is a chronic vascular disease of unknown cause, which is characterized by progressive inflammation of the cranial arteries, often with giant cells and granulomas. The disease is somewhat more common in elderly women than in elderly men and is an important cause of blindness in this age-group. Early symptoms include headache and jaw pain upon chewing or speaking. Later, there is decline in vision, usually in one eye but occasionally in both eyes. The diagnosis of giant cell arteritis is aided by measurement of the erythrocyte sedimentation rate, which is elevated in most cases. Definitive diagnosis is made by temporal artery biopsy; arteriography is not as useful for the diagnosis because of low sensitivity and frequent false-positive results. The treatment of choice is prednisone, which should be started as soon as giant cell arteritis is suspected. Without prompt and thorough treatment, irreversible blindness can occur.

9. The answer is C. Multicenter collaborative studies of acute herpes simplex virus-1 (HSV-1) encephalitis have established many facts about the nature of this disease. The disease has no gender or age predilection and exhibits no seasonal fluctuations in incidence. Although the exact pathogenesis in adults is unclear, temporal lobe viral spread from trigeminal or olfactory nerves is likely, often due to reactivation of latent virus. Also, it has been shown that HSV-1 encephalitis usually does not occur in association with active herpes infection at other body sites. Data from these studies indicate that electroencephalography provides early supportive information more often than CT or nuclear brain scanning. CSF examination and culture cannot provide valuable diagnostic information; the findings (e.g., the presence of erythrocytes) are nonspecific, and the culture results usually are negative. At present, the diagnosis is best established by brain biopsy and culture, although new techniques are being tested. One of these is MRI to identify early stages of HSV-1 encephalitis; this procedure may become the most sensitive, noninvasive test for early diagnosis.

10. The answer is D. Normal pressure hydrocephalus (also called communicating hydrocephalus) is an imprecise term used to refer to a disorder of ventricular enlargement with normal CSF pressure and a characteristic presentation of broad-based ataxic gait, dementia, and urinary incontinence. A variety of disorders are included in the differential diagnosis of normal pressure hydrocephalus by virtue of their association with ventricular enlargement, abnormal gait, memory loss, or incontinence. In Alzheimer's disease, a gait disorder exists but is insignificant in comparison to the profound loss of memory; this plus the presence of aphasia allows for a diagnosis of Alzheimer's disease over normal pressure hydrocephalus. The absence of urinary incontinence and the presence of tremor and rigidity distinguish Parkinson's disease from normal pressure hydrocephalus. A broad-based gait would likely characterize alcohol-related cerebellar disease and memory impairment might arise from more generalized cerebral effects of alcohol, but upper extremity involvement and the usual absence of urinary disturbances would help to distinguish this disorder. Multi-infarct dementia, although potentially similar to normal pressure hydrocephalus in its presentation, usually can be ruled out by CT scanning, which shows multiple brain infarcts. Although depression may present as pseudodementia, careful mental status testing can distinguish depression from true dementia; gait disturbances and incontinence are not features of depression.

11. The answer is B. Chronic symptomatic (normal pressure) hydrocephalus in the elderly most often is caused by head trauma or spontaneous subarachnoid hemorrhage. Patients typically present with a progressive dementia as well as an ataxic gait and urinary incontinence. Ventricular shunting has been used to treat these patients; however, not all patients with large ventricles respond to a shunting procedure and selection of patients often is difficult. In general, the response to shunting seems to be better when a definite cause can be identified and there has been a relatively short duration of the full syndrome. The absence of cerebral atrophy on CT and temporary psychomotor improvement following drainage by lumbar puncture are other factors that appear to correlate with a better shunt outcome.

12. The answer is B. The syndrome of parkinsonism usually is caused by an idiopathic degenerative disorder of the basal ganglia (referred to as paralysis agitans, or Parkinson's disease). Parkinsonism also may result from exposure to certain neurotoxic substances, antipsychotic drugs, and certain metabolic disorders (e.g., Wilson's disease). The cardinal features of parkinsonism include a rhythmic resting tremor (pill-rolling tremor), generalized slowness of movement (bradykinesia), muscle rigidity with resistance to passive movement (cogwheel rigidity), disorders of posture, and festinating gait. In addition, advanced cases may include mild dementia and depression. Dysmetria refers to a disturbance in one's ability to control the range of movement in a muscular action; dysmetria is not a feature of parkinsonism but is a sign of cerebellar disease.

13. The answer is B. Parkinsonism may be combined with other neurologic disorders in what are called "parkinsonism-plus" syndromes. Some of the more common defects found with parkinsonism include progressive supranuclear palsy, autonomic dysfunction (Shy-Drager syndrome), dementia, normal pressure hydrocephalus, and hereditary disorders such as Wilson's disease and Huntington's disease; seizures are no more common in patients with Parkinson's disease than in the general population, and no specific designation is given to the combination of these defects. Shy-Drager syndrome refers to an idiopathic disorder characterized by progressive deterioration in autonomic function combined with degeneration elsewhere in the CNS. The basic lesion is a loss of neurons, especially in the intermediolateral columns (the site of preganglionic sympathetic neurons), but also in the substantia nigra, cerebellum, and striatum. Shy-Drager syndrome typically presents in middle age (between the ages of 40 and 60 years) and is more common in men. Early manifestations of autonomic insufficiency, such as anhidrosis, sphincter disturbances, and impotence, may be ignored; however, there is progression to more incapacitating features, notably severe postural hypotension. Neurologic signs reflect the involvement of the substantia nigra (which produces parkinsonism), the cerebellum (which produces ataxia), and striatum (which results in a lack of response to levodopa). Shy-Drager syndrome is relatively unchanged by treatment, although postural hypotension may be improved by drug therapy.

14. The answer is B. Several studies have documented the association between amaurosis fugax (transient monocular blindness) and ipsilateral atherosclerotic carotid artery disease. Patients who present with this symptom (usually described as being similar to having a shade pulled down over one's eye) should be considered for carotid artery diagnostic studies, which detect carotid disease in nearly half of cases. Regardless of this, it is important to rule out giant cell (temporal) arteritis in an elderly patient who suddenly loses vision in one eye, as this disorder can lead to permanent blindness if not promptly treated with corticosteroids. In most cases, giant cell arteritis can be identified by an elevated erythrocyte sedimentation rate found in association with typical symptoms such as headache or jaw claudication. The other disorders listed in the question do not produce amaurosis fugax, although other visual defects may occur. Pseudotumor cerebri most frequently causes problems with visual field constriction, retinal detachment is associated with sparkling and "floaters," migraine usually presents as transient visual field cuts, and pituitary adenoma causes bitemporal hemianopia that is progressive with increasing size of the tumor.

15. The answer is E. Meige's syndrome (blepharospasm, oromandibular dystonia) is one of the most common focal torsion dystonias of adulthood. Typically, the onset of symptoms is in middle age, beginning as periodic episodes of increased blinking (blepharospasm), which often is aggravated by bright lights. Over time, the spasms become more intense and more frequent, eventually involving the muscles of the entire face (especially around the lips) and the jaw muscles. In severe cases, the blepharospasm can cause functional blindness. Surgical therapy often can relieve the dystonia; drug therapy, however, has not proven to be effective. Low-dose injections of botulinum toxin into the eyelid muscles can alleviate the blepharospasm temporarily. This treatment, performed 3 or 4 times per year, is useful for elderly persons who cannot undergo surgery.

16. The answer is C. Syncope refers to a sudden temporary loss of consciousness and postural tone, which most frequently is due to an acute generalized decrease in cerebral blood flow. Vasodepressor (vasovagal) causes of syncope are common in all age-groups, especially the young; a surge in the activity of the cholinergic nervous system causes sudden massive venodilation and fainting due to decreased cardiac preload. Vasodepressor syncope often is due to psychological or emotional effects on the autonomic nervous system.

Normal aging is associated with certain physiologic changes that, when combined with the effects of particular drugs or disorders, can lead to an interruption of cerebral blood flow and syncope. Two causes of syncope that are more common in the elderly are orthostatic (postural) hypotension and arrhythmias. Elderly persons are particularly prone to orthostatic hypotension, which may occur due to several factors. In Shy-Drager syndrome, progressive deterioration of the autonomic nervous system produces severe orthostatic hypotension. Diabetes, a fairly frequent disease of the elderly, may produce peripheral neuropathy, with subsequent autonomic nervous system deficiency producing orthostatic hypotension. Certain drugs commonly used by elderly patients also can produce orthostatic hypotension by blocking the sympathetic nervous system; examples include amitryptyline (a tricyclic antidepressant), methyldopa (an antihypertensive), and phenothiazines. Diuretics and nitrates may produce orthostatic hypotension by other mechanisms.

A variety of arrhythmias and conduction disturbances may produce syncope, primarily by causing a decrease in left ventricular output. In comparison to orthostatic hypotension and arrhythmias, COPD is very unlikely to cause syncope except in rare instances of chronic bronchitis, as a result of severe and repeated coughing. Vertebrobasilar insufficiency may be associated with sudden loss of postural tone ("drop attacks") but without loss of consciousness, and epilepsy may present with sudden loss of consciousness that should be distinguished from syncope.

17. The answer is A. Disorders of movement (tremor, gait disturbances) are common signs of age-related changes in neurologic function. The tremor seen most frequently in elderly persons is an action tremor sometimes referred to as senile tremor, although a more appropriate term is essential tremor. Typically, essential tremor begins in later life and is most significant in parts of the body that maintain posture; the tremor is amplified with activity and reduced upon relaxation of the limbs or body parts affected. In contrast, the tremor of Parkinson's disease usually is a resting tremor; that is, the tremor disappears when the affected limb or body part is used. Although Parkinson's disease is primarily a disease of elderly persons and drug-induced parkinsonism also is a problem, parkinsonian tremor is not as frequent as essential tremor. Cerebellar disease also can produce a tremor (often confused with essential tremor), which is characterized by a variable rate seen only on movement as well as dysmetria. Cerebellar tremor is an uncommon clinical manifestation that would be restricted to cases of midline cerebellar disease due to alcoholism, cerebellar stroke, or malignancy. Patients with significant hyperthyroidism (thyrotoxicosis) frequently develop a tremor similar to the exaggerated physiologic tremor produced in hyperadrenergic states; however, this is not as likely as essential tremor.

18. The answer is D. Chronic subdural hematoma usually follows mild rather than severe head injury and is most common in men who are chronic alcoholics and in the elderly; spontaneous subdural hematoma may occur in patients on long-term anticoagulation or dialysis. Symptoms may not develop until days or weeks after the injury and typically begin with headache followed by intermittent confusion, drowsiness, and obtundation. Eventually, lateralizing neurologic signs (e.g., hemiparesis, hemianopia) may occur, although these are not consistent findings. Angiography no longer is necessary to make the diagnosis; CT and MRI scanning are sufficient. In some cases, small hematomas resolve spontaneously. Large hematomas usually require surgical drainage.

19. The answer is D. Amyotrophic lateral sclerosis is a relentlessly progressive disease characterized by degeneration of the pyramidal motor neurons in the cortex, brain stem, and anterior horns of the spinal cord. Both upper and lower motor neurons are affected. The onset of amyotrophic lateral sclerosis typically is between the ages of 40 and 60 years, and death within 5 years is common; men are affected twice as often as women. The disease has a variety of manifestations. Usually, weakness develops in the hands and progresses upward to the shoulders and cranial musculature. Aching of the muscles is common, but sensory findings are absent, as are bladder and bowel dysfunction. Vision also is unaffected. Patients may present with pseudobulbar palsy early in the course of the disease and, thus, may experience uncontrollable laughing and crying. The hallmark of amyotrophic lateral sclerosis is fasciculations of the muscles (of the hands and arms, especially). Hyperreflexia and muscle wasting also are characteristic.

20. The answer is A. Cervical spondylosis is a disorder of unknown cause, although advancing age, diabetes mellitus, and trauma appear to be associated with its development. The disorder leads to osteophyte formation and narrowing of the intervertebral spaces, with resultant nerve root compression; spinal cord compression also may occur in persons with a congenitally narrow spinal canal. Symptoms typically develop insidiously in late adulthood, beginning with neck pain and radicular pain combined with weakness, fasciculations, areflexia, and sensory loss of the upper extremities. The disorder rarely is symmetrical. Involvement of the lower extremities occurs later, with increased tendon reflexes, decreased sensations, and a slow, stiff gait. Conservative treatment (e.g., with cervical collar and traction) is appropriate for patients with less severe symptoms. Surgery is recommended for patients with serious neurologic impairment to arrest the myelopathic progression.

21. The answer is C. Several factors have been shown to affect significantly the prognosis for a patient who has suffered a stroke. Chief among these is the age of the patient (the mortality rate is much greater in patients over age 70), the presence of underlying disease (especially hypertension, cardiovascular disease, or diabetes mellitus), the degree of neurologic deficit (sensory loss and hemiplegia are poor prognostic signs), and the degree of consciousness (coma suggests a poor prognosis). There is only minimal evidence that the particular artery involved in a stroke influences the prognosis; patients who have had strokes involving the vertebrobasilar system have a slightly better prognosis than patients whose first stroke involved the carotid circulation.

22. The answer is E. The history and physical examination of this patient do not suggest the need for any of the diagnostic procedures listed; lumbar puncture, x-ray, electromyography, and Doppler studies all are inappropriate or too expensive. The complaint of diminished strength is a common clinical manifestation, which may result from a variety of neurologic or muscular disorders. The diagnosis of Parkinson's disease is one of exclusion, but it is too soon to begin expensive testing.

23. The answer is D. This patient clearly manifests certain cardinal features of Parkinson's disease (tremor, rigidity), which are predominantly unilateral in presentation, although there is evidence of some bilateral involvement. These symptoms, although embarrassing, are not severe enough to require strong antiparkinsonian agents such as levodopa or bromocriptine. The best therapeutic course at this stage of Parkinson's disease is to begin treatment with a weak antiparkinsonian agent, the weakest of which is trihexyphenidyl (an anticholinergic agent). If the patient does not show enough improvement on anticholinergic medication, amantadine should be tried instead, as it is better to start a patient on one drug at a time. Both amantadine and anticholinergic agents are very useful as adjuvant agents later in the disease, to enhance the therapeutic benefit from levodopa.

24. The answer is A. The history and physical examination of this patient are most compatible with a peripheral nerve injury—carpal tunnel syndrome. Tapping over the median nerve at the wrist may elicit electric sensations in the hand (Tinel's sign), and holding the wrist plantar-flexed at 90° may elicit numbness (Phalen's sign). Although carotid bruits are present and cervical spine arthritis is suggested, the pathophysiologic features appear to be most consistent with a chronic entrapment syndrome. Electromyelography and nerve conduction velocity (EMG/NCV) studies should provide evidence of delayed nerve conduction at the wrist. X-rays of the cervical spine, hand, and wrist are unlikely to be helpful. Although carotid bruits are present, noninvasive carotid studies would not be useful for evaluating a peripheral entrapment syndrome.

25. The answer is B. This patient demonstrates only sensory findings of carpal tunnel syndrome, which probably can be managed conservatively with resting wrist splints, nonsteroidal anti-inflammatory drugs, or corticosteroid injections into the carpal tunnel. Surgical decompression would be definitive therapy, but this treatment usually is reserved for intractable complaints or demonstrable motor involvement. Systemic corticosteroids would be of no benefit in treatment of this patient's carpal tunnel syndrome.

26. The answer is E. Carpal tunnel syndrome may be associated with a variety of disorders. The median nerve is compressed at the wrist when there is wrist infiltration by amyloid, tophaceous deposits (in gout), or mucinous deposits (in diabetes or hypothyroidism). Tenosynovitis of the wrist tendons can occur in persons with chronic inflammatory conditions (e.g., rheumatoid arthritis) or can result from manual labor that is performed by a person who is unaccustomed to such strenuous activity. To the extent that a reversible cause can be demonstrated and treated, surgery to transect the transverse carpal ligament may be avoided. However, surgery usually is needed when the carpal tunnel is affected by an infiltrative process. Osteoporosis is not a cause of carpal tunnel syndrome.

27–30. The answers are: 27-T, 28-T, 29-F, 30-F. A transient ischemic attack (TIA) is a focal disturbance of cerebral function that typically has an abrupt onset and a rapid recovery with no residual neurologic deficits. TIAs develop most commonly in persons between the ages of 60 and 70 years. Although spontaneous remission does occur, more often TIAs tend to recur and, more importantly, lead to stroke. Recognizing and treating the cause of TIAs, therefore, is the best means of preventing stroke.

Most TIAs are believed to result from thromboembolism originating in the extracranial carotid artery. Whenever possible, an attempt should be made to distinguish between TIAs that occur in carotid arteries and TIAs that occur in the vertebrobasilar circulation, as the clinical course is more aggressive in carotid artery disease; carotid TIAs lead to stroke sooner and after fewer attacks than vertebrobasilar TIAs. Symptoms that develop during an attack often suggest the location of the ischemia.

The symptom that is most suggestive of carotid disease is amaurosis fugax (transient monocular blindness), which results from retinal ischemia. Carotid TIAs also may be due to cerebral hemisphere ischemia (rarely at the same time as retinal ischemia), which produces hemiparesis or monoparesis and localized tingling and numbness; loss of consciousness rarely occurs in carotid TIAs, and transient global amnesia never occurs.

The symptoms of vertebrobasilar disease are more varied. The most frequent feature is vertigo, followed by diplopia and binocular visual disturbances (ranging from dimness to total blindness). Involvement of the long motor and sensory tracts produces sensorimotor disturbances on one or both sides of the body. It is believed that most cases of transient global amnesia (a syndrome that most commonly affects older men) are related to vertebrobasilar ischemia. Drop attacks also are characteristic of vertebrobasilar insufficiency. These attacks involve a sudden loss of postural tone due to weakness in the antigravity muscles; there is no loss of consciousness, however.

31–34. The answers are: 31-F, 32-T, 33-F, 34-T. Parkinsonism, although most frequently an idiopathic disorder, can be induced by exposure to certain toxic substances, including drugs administered for psychotic illness. The parkinsonian syndrome that can develop with chronic ingestion of antipsychotic medications may be indistinguishable from idiopathic parkinsonism and nearly as common.

Antipsychotic agents induce parkinsonism by blocking dopamine$_2$ (D_2) receptors on postsynaptic neurons in the striatum, not by depleting dopamine storage sites (the mechanism by which reserpine induces parkinsonism). Patients receiving these drugs are at greatest risk for developing the syndrome within the first 30 days of antipsychotic therapy. Rigidity and resting tremor are the most prominent features, although bradykinesia and masked facies also may be noted.

Treatment with levodopa does not reverse the syndrome because the dopamine receptors are already occupied by the antipsychotic drug. However, anticholinergic agents are effective. Withdrawal of the antipsychotic drug leads to eventual clearing of all neurologic effects, although this may take months.

Notable other causes of secondary parkinsonism include intoxication by carbon monoxide or manganese. Recently, an association of parkinsonism with the synthetic meperidine analogue, MPTP, has been noted in drug addicts and chemists who have been exposed to the substance.

35–38. The answers are: 35-F, 36-T, 37-T, 38-F. Progressive supranuclear palsy (also known as Steele-Richardson-Olszewski syndrome) is the most common of the "parkinsonism-plus" syndromes. The disorder involves neuronal loss and neurofibrillary tangles in the basal ganglia, brain stem, and cerebellum. No effective treatment is known.

Progressive supranuclear palsy can resemble Parkinson's disease clinically. Patients present with gait ataxia and postural instability resulting in frequent falls. Tremor is unusual, however. Other distinguishing features include nuchal and facial dystonia and unresponsiveness to levodopa.

The most distinguishing feature of progressive supranuclear palsy, however, is the lack of voluntary eye movement (ophthalmoplegia). Whereas Parkinson's disease also is characterized by impaired upward gaze and convergence, progressive supranuclear palsy can be identified by the added features of impaired downward and lateral gaze. The clinical picture may not include all of these oculomotor disorders until late in the course of the disease. In such cases, a tentative diagnosis of progressive supranuclear palsy is made on the basis of the other features that distinguish it from Parkinson's disease.

39–42. The answers are: 39-T, 40-F, 41-F, 42-T. In the absence of evidence to suggest orthostatic hypotension or vasodepressor stimuli as the cause of this patient's syncopal episodes, it is appropriate to evaluate for cardiac causes to explain these symptoms. Although not as common as orthostatic or vasodepressor mechanisms, cardiogenic mechanisms of syncope often reflect serious heart disease and, thus, should be sought.

Serum electrolyte evaluation is indicated for this patient, especially to uncover an abnormally high or low serum potassium level, which can predispose to cardiac arrhythmias and syncope. Prolonged electrocardiographic (Holter) monitoring also is indicated to identify an occult rhythm disturbance, which, because of the episodic nature of arrhythmias, may be missed by a single electrocardiographic evaluation. Holter monitoring may not uncover all arrhythmias and conduction blocks but usually is sufficient to make a diagnosis in a patient with syncope. Brain scanning, CT scanning, skull x-ray, and electroencephalography rarely provide useful information in the absence of neurologic signs and symptoms and are unnecessarily costly.

43–46. The answers are: 43-T, 44-T, 45-T, 46-F. Physicians who care for older patients frequently must distinguish true muscle weakness from fatigue or tiredness.

Guillain-Barré syndrome is an idiopathic disorder believed to be autoimmune in nature, which is characterized by progressive paralysis beginning in the feet and ascending upward. The condition may occur at any age and usually has an acute onset. An antecedent event, usually a gastrointestinal or upper respiratory infection 1–8 weeks prior to the onset of weakness, is documented in most cases. Swallowing difficulty and impaired breathing are the most serious symptoms of Guillain-Barré syndrome.

Myasthenia gravis is a disorder of neuromuscular function believed to be caused by the presence of antibodies to acetylcholine receptors at the neuromuscular junction. Typically, myasthenia gravis causes transient attacks of fatigue and weakness in certain muscle groups, most commonly those innervated by the cranial nerves, although severe generalized weakness may occur. Persons of all ages may be affected. Among adults, the incidence in women is highest in early adulthood and in men is highest in the sixth decade.

Polymyositis is an idiopathic inflammatory muscle disease; an autoimmune mechanism may play a role in its development. Typically, patients present with symmetrical, proximal, upper and lower extremity muscle weakness that is steadily progressive. The disease is somewhat rare, with bimodal peaks in incidence (childhood and late adulthood).

Polymyalgia rheumatica is a syndrome of muscle and joint stiffness and aching, predominantly in the shoulder and hip girdles, which occurs only in people over 50 years of age. True muscle weakness rarely is present in this disorder.

47–50. The answers are: 47-F, 48-T, 49-F, 50-F. In 1986, the National Conference on Antithrombotic Therapy (NCAT) established guidelines for the use of anticoagulants in patients at risk for the onset, or worsening, of stroke.

Patients who experience transient ischemic attacks (TIAs) have a 10% annual risk of completed stroke or death. According to NCAT, the risk of stroke and death is reduced significantly with aspirin in a dosage of 1 g/day. Anticoagulants, however, show no clear benefit in this situation. Given the known risk of hemorrhagic side effects with anticoagulation, these agents are not recommended for patients with TIAs.

A progressing thrombotic stroke refers to a focal neurologic impairment that worsens progressively (from minutes to days) after its presentation. Many patients with thrombotic stroke exhibit such a progression. According to NCAT, anticoagulants are favored for prevention of a deteriorating condition and death in patients who have documented absence of hemorrhage.

A completed thrombotic stroke refers to a focal neurologic impairment that has remained stable for 24 hours. According to NCAT, anticoagulants show no benefit and can be harmful in this situation. Aspirin, however, clearly benefited patients with completed strokes.

According to NCAT, anticoagulants are not recommended for the prevention of stroke in patients with endocarditis of a native heart valve.

7
Musculoskeletal Disorders

QUESTIONS

Directions: Each question below contains five suggested answers. Choose the **one best** response to each question.

1. Which of the following statements regarding aging muscle tissue is true?

(A) The density of capillaries per motor unit remains unchanged
(B) The oxygen utilization per unit of tissue decreases
(C) Muscle contraction time shortens
(D) Myosin ATPase activity is unchanged
(E) The number of muscle cells decreases

2. Many disorders that involve the joints reflect a defect in the immune system. The most basic deficit in immune function that occurs with aging is a decrease in

(A) the functional activity of T cells
(B) the functional activity of B cells
(C) polymorphonuclear migration
(D) macrophage phagocytosis
(E) monocyte chemotaxis

3. Clinical manifestations of osteoarthritis include all of the following EXCEPT

(A) prolonged periods of stiffness
(B) enlarged joints
(C) flexion contractures
(D) radiographic evidence of joint space narrowing
(E) calcium pyrophosphate dihydrate crystals in the synovial fluid

4. Rheumatoid arthritis is characterized by all of the following radiographic findings EXCEPT

(A) bone erosion
(B) soft tissue swelling
(C) joint space narrowing
(D) juxta-articular demineralization
(E) osteophytes

5. Which of the following findings is definitive evidence of calcium pyrophosphate dihydrate deposition disease as the cause of an acute inflammatory arthritis?

(A) Negatively birefringent, needle-shaped crystals on microscopic examination of the synovial fluid
(B) Chondrocalcinosis on radiographic examination of the involved joint
(C) Extensive osteophytes on radiographic examination of the involved joint
(D) Positively birefringent, rectangular crystals on microscopic examination of the synovial fluid
(E) Large numbers of neutrophils in the synovial fluid

6. The screening evaluation of an elderly patient with a vertebral compression fracture and radiographic evidence of osteopenia should include all of the following tests EXCEPT

(A) thyroid function testing
(B) measurement of 24-hour urine hydroxyproline excretion
(C) overnight dexamethasone suppression testing
(D) serum chemistry screening
(E) serum protein electrophoresis

7. Fibrositis is a syndrome characterized by generalized aching and specific sites of localized tenderness. In its primary form, fibrositis usually appears in the teenage years and may be a lifelong problem. When it appears later in life, fibrositis often is the initial manifestation of an underlying disorder. Late-onset fibrositis can be associated with all of the following disorders EXCEPT

(A) rheumatoid arthritis
(B) osteomalacia
(C) hypothyroidism
(D) depression
(E) Alzheimer's disease

8. The most common presentation of calcium pyrophosphate dihydrate deposition in the elderly is

(A) pseudogout
(B) pseudo–rheumatoid arthritis
(C) asymptomatic calcification found on x-ray
(D) periarticular inflammation
(E) Milwaukee shoulder

9. Patients with rheumatoid arthritis may exhibit all of the following extra-articular manifestations of disease EXCEPT

(A) nodules
(B) vasculitis
(C) interstitial lung disease
(D) anterior uveitis
(E) thrombocytosis

10. All of the following statements concerning elderly-onset systemic lupus erythematosus are true EXCEPT

(A) the incidence is equal in men and women
(B) elderly patients often present with symptomatic pleuritis or pericarditis
(C) the prognosis is better than that for younger patients
(D) renal involvement is common
(E) lupus pneumonitis and pulmonary fibrosis are more common than in younger patients

11. All of the following statements describe hydroxyapatite arthropathy EXCEPT

(A) it is associated with degenerative joint disease
(B) the shoulder and knee are the most commonly involved joints
(C) joint fluids typically are inflammatory
(D) destructive joint and tendon findings are common
(E) it is also called Milwaukee shoulder

12. An 85-year-old woman complains of an aching, burning pain in the right lateral hip area, which radiates along the front of the thigh to the knee and which is especially acute when she crosses the affected leg over the other leg. She says the pain is worse when she walks, and it restricts her from lying on her right side at night. The most likely cause of this patient's symptoms is

(A) osteoarthritis of the hip
(B) avascular necrosis of the hip
(C) trochanteric bursitis
(D) meralgia paresthetica
(E) sciatica

13. Elderly patients with rheumatoid arthritis may require treatment with a disease-modifying agent such as gold. Good reasons for beginning treatment with one of these drugs include all of the following EXCEPT

(A) persistent polyarticular synovitis
(B) progressive deformities
(C) radiographic evidence of erosive joint disease
(D) chronic joint pain
(E) failure to respond to nonsteroidal anti-inflammatory drugs

14. Isolated angiitis of the CNS occurs most commonly in middle-aged and elderly persons, and its clinical effects often are confused with those of atherosclerosis or hypertension. Which of the following clinical features most strongly suggests that isolated CNS angiitis is the cause of new focal neurologic defects rather than a more common cause of cerebrovascular disease?

(A) A history of persistent, severe headache and altered mental status
(B) Funduscopic evidence of retinal microaneurysms and hemorrhage
(C) Arthralgias and myalgias
(D) High-titer positive antinuclear antibody
(E) Mild peripheral neuropathy

15. An overweight elderly woman complains of mild right knee pain. She claims that she cannot sleep with her knees touching and has to put a pillow between her legs. She notes that her right leg feels stiff upon awakening but usually feels better once she has been moving around for a few minutes. Examination of the right knee reveals bone hypertrophy and mild varus deformity. This constellation of symptoms and signs is most suggestive of

(A) pes anserine bursitis
(B) medial compartment degenerative joint disease
(C) patellar–femoral degenerative joint disease
(D) avascular necrosis of the medial tibial plateau
(E) popliteal cyst

16. Which of the following findings is suggestive of secondary, rather than primary, Sjögren's syndrome?

(A) Keratoconjunctivitis sicca
(B) Positive lip biopsy (lymphocytic infiltration of minor salivary glands)
(C) Peripheral neuropathy
(D) Erosive arthritis
(E) Xerostomia

17. An elderly patient is being considered for total hip replacement for severe degenerative joint disease. All of the following factors have an important effect on surgical risk EXCEPT

(A) age of 85 years
(B) serum albumin of 2.7 g/dl
(C) prior unstable angina
(D) moderate obstructive defect on pulmonary function testing
(E) systolic blood pressure of 160/100 mm Hg

18. Which of the following factors is the most significant contraindication to total knee replacement?

(A) Moderate rather than severe radiographic changes of osteoarthritis
(B) Pronounced varus deformity
(C) Joint ankylosis
(D) Existing rheumatoid arthritis
(E) History of thrombophlebitis

19. A 65-year-old patient with progressive rheumatoid arthritis is no longer benefiting from the administration of nonsteroidal anti-inflammatory agents, and auranofin is prescribed. All of the following statements about auranofin are true EXCEPT

(A) it may be somewhat less effective than injectable gold for the treatment of rheumatoid arthritis
(B) it is more likely than injectable gold to cause renal or mucocutaneous toxicity
(C) a high incidence of diarrhea is associated with its use
(D) eosinophilia and proteinuria often occur with its use
(E) cutaneous reactions often are seen

20. Amyloidosis is a term for several disorders, all of which are characterized by accumulation of insoluble proteins (amyloid fibrils) in organs. Which of the following statements is true about one of these disorders—senile amyloidosis?

(A) The disorder involves the deposition of immunoglobulin light chains
(B) Myocardial function is relatively preserved even with extensive infiltration
(C) Most patients die as a result of cardiac arrhythmias
(D) The kidney is the most commonly involved organ
(E) The diagnosis is made best by rectal or skin biopsy

21. In the geriatric population, the occurrence of polymyositis in association with cancer is best characterized by which of the following statements?

(A) Polymyositis is more likely than dermatomyositis to be associated with malignancy
(B) The malignancies that commonly are associated with polymyositis are those that are common in the general elderly population
(C) Polymyositis that occurs with malignancy is likely to be associated with vasculitis as well
(D) Removal of an associated tumor usually cures the polymyositis
(E) A screening evaluation for cancer is unnecessary in elderly-onset polymyositis

22. Polymyalgia rheumatica commonly is associated with all of the following clinical features EXCEPT

(A) muscle weakness
(B) low-grade fever
(C) mild synovitis
(D) anemia
(E) elevated serum alkaline phosphatase level

Directions: The groups of questions below consist of an introductory premise or case data followed by four statements that pertain to the information given. Indicate whether each statement is **true** or **false**.

Questions 23–26

Urate deposition in tissues of gout patients can be reversed with administration of the following drugs.

23. Colchicine
24. Allopurinol
25. Indomethacin
26. Probenecid

Questions 27–30

Definitive treatment of gout involves chronic administration of drugs that reduce serum uric acid levels. Chronic drug therapy would be indicated in the following elderly patients with hyperuricemia.

27. An 86-year-old woman with impaired renal function
28. A 76-year-old man with recurrent attacks of acute gout
29. A 78-year-old man with tophaceous gout
30. A 75-year-old man with a history of urolithiasis

Questions 31–34

Appropriate treatments for vertebral compression fractures include the following.

31. Bed rest and pain relief
32. Corset
33. Truncal casting
34. Surgical fixation

Questions 35–38

The side effects of nonsteroidal anti-inflammatory drugs (NSAIDs) are important causes of morbidity in the elderly. The following are appropriate guidelines for the safe use of NSAIDs in elderly patients.

35. The administration of indomethacin with triamterene is unsafe
36. The use of ibuprofen in a patient with asthma, nasal polyps, and aspirin sensitivity generally is safe
37. Ibuprofen is less likely than aspirin to cause gastrointestinal toxicity
38. Nonacetylated salicylates can be used safely in patients taking anticoagulants

Questions 39–42

The following statements describe risk factors for hip fracture in the elderly.

39. The risk of fracture is greater with type I involutional osteoporosis (associated with low or normal levels of PTH) than with type II involutional osteoporosis (associated with high levels of PTH)
40. The use of antipsychotic drugs increases the risk of fracture
41. Obese persons are at a greater risk for fracture than lean persons
42. Blacks with osteoporosis are less likely than whites to suffer hip fracture

Questions 43–46

All of the elderly patients described below have potential clinical evidence of giant cell (temporal) arteritis.

43. A 65-year-old woman who complains of fatigue and poor memory

44. A 90-year-old man who complains of aching in the back of his head and generalized stiffness in his shoulders and thighs, which have persisted for 1 month

45. An 82-year-old man who has just noted the sensation of a curtain coming down over his left eye, which resolved completely within 15 minutes

46. A confused 65-year-old woman with a history of hard-to-control diabetes and hypertension who is brought to the emergency room with a blood pressure of 240/140 mm Hg; funduscopic evidence of papilledema, hemorrhage, and cotton-wool spots; and bilateral basilar rales

Questions 47–50

The incidence of osteoarthritis increases with age. The following are true statements about the epidemiology of osteoarthritis.

47. Osteoarthritis primarily is an asymptomatic, polyarticular disease

48. The particular joint sites affected by osteoarthritis vary with gender and race

49. The incidence of osteoarthritis increases with increased physical activity

50. The incidence of osteoarthritis is increased in patients with diabetes mellitus or hemochromatosis

Questions 51–54

An elderly woman complains that for several months she has had intermittent redness, swelling, and stiffness in the distal interphalangeal joints of her hands. She has no other joint or systemic complaints. The following diagnoses should be considered.

51. Erosive osteoarthritis

52. Rheumatoid arthritis

53. Psoriatic arthritis

54. Ankylosing spondylitis

ANSWERS AND EXPLANATIONS

1. The answer is E. Many changes occur in human muscle tissue that are related to the aging process. Progressive loss of strength is a generalized finding that is associated with specific age-related changes, including a reduction in the capillary density per motor unit. Although oxygen utilization per unit of tissue remains largely unchanged, myosin ATPase activity decreases, which correlates with a lengthening of muscle contraction time and a decrease in the maximal rate of tension development. The total number of muscle cells declines linearly with age, but the generalized muscle atrophy may go unnoticed because of increased interstitial fluid, fat, and collagen.

2. The answer is A. Thymic involution and decreased functional activity of T cells are the major changes in immune function that occur with aging. Impaired cell-mediated immunity consequent to these changes is reflected in an increasing prevalence of cutaneous anergy. Functional B cell changes (e.g., decreased antibody production with age, decreased antibody response to administered vaccines) are secondary to the T cell deficit. Polymorphonuclear migration remains intact, but chemotaxis may be slightly reduced. There are no consistent changes in macrophage or monocyte function.

3. The answer is A. Signs and symptoms of osteoarthritis are well-defined. Pain usually is described as a generalized aching, which is worsened with activity and improved with rest. Rather than prolonged periods of stiffness, the disease is characterized by brief periods (about 30 minutes) of morning stiffness and stiffness after rest (the so-called gelling phenomenon). Range of motion is reduced as the disease advances, and the involved joints become enlarged. This latter finding is the result of periarticular bone enlargement and, occasionally, small noninflammatory effusions. Radiography usually reveals joint space narrowing as well as subchondral bone sclerosis, pseudocysts, and marginal osteophytes. Calcium pyrophosphate dihydrate crystals and calcium hydroxyapatite crystals can be found in synovial effusions in patients with osteoarthritis. The prevalence of these crystals increases with the severity of the degenerative joint disease.

4. The answer is E. Radiographic evidence of rheumatoid arthritis may be absent early in the disease process. Soft tissue swelling around distended joints may be detected early, although this finding is more easily noted on physical examination. Juxta-articular osteopenia can occur relatively early (within months after the onset of disease) and may parallel disease activity. Bone erosions occur first at the joint margins, in the so-called "bare areas," where synovium is reflected over bone and not cartilage. Joint space narrowing is a sign of cartilage loss and, in rheumatoid arthritis, involves the entire joint; in osteoarthritis, narrowing more commonly occurs in only one area of the joint, especially in weight-bearing joints (e.g., medial compartment loss in knee osteoarthritis). Osteophytes, subchondral bone sclerosis, and subchondral cyst formation all are radiographic features of osteoarthritis.

5. The answer is D. Inflammatory calcium pyrophosphate dihydrate (CPPD) deposition disease, or pseudogout, is a particularly common cause of inflammatory arthritis in the elderly because of the high incidence of CPPD deposition disease in this population. The best evidence that pseudogout is the cause of an acute arthritis is the finding of chunky, rhomboid or rectangular crystals that exhibit positive birefringence in red-compensated, polarized light on microscopic examination of synovial fluid. Chondrocalcinosis on x-ray of the involved joint certainly is suggestive evidence of CPPD deposition; however, this finding is so common in some elderly populations that it may be misleading. The finding of large numbers of neutrophils in the synovial fluid suggests only an inflammatory arthritis, not a specific cause. Negatively birefringent, needle-shaped crystals are urate crystals—the synovial fluid finding in gout. Osteophytes mark the presence of osteoarthritis, either primary or secondary.

6. The answer is B. The measurement of 24-hour urine hydroxyproline excretion is useful as an index of bone collagen resorption. This test typically is used to measure disease activity in Paget's disease but not to screen for a cause of osteopenia. When evaluating a patient who has experienced a vertebral fracture due to osteopenia, it is essential to consider not only primary osteoporosis and secondary causes of osteoporosis but also diseases that mimic osteoporosis.

The history and physical examination should aim to uncover factors that might be associated with osteopenia, such as dietary deficiencies (e.g., of calcium or vitamin D), drug intake (e.g., use of phenytoin or barbiturates, which is associated with osteomalacia), and certain systemic disorders (e.g., intestinal malabsorption, metastatic cancer, systemic mastocytosis). Laboratory testing should include routine serum chemistry screening, since a low calcium or phosphorus level and an elevated alkaline phosphatase level suggest the diagnosis of osteomalacia.

Routine screening for hyperthyroidism with thyroid function testing and for adrenocortical excess with overnight dexamethasone suppression testing also are indicated, because findings on history and physical examination may be subtle even with widespread osteoporosis. Serum protein electrophoresis, urine protein electrophoresis, CBC, and erythrocyte sedimentation rate are adequate screening tests for multiple myeloma if all results are normal.

Evaluation of serum 25-hydroxycholecalciferol and 24-hour urine calcium levels also is useful in distinguishing between osteoporosis and osteomalacia. If osteomalacia still cannot be ruled out and treatment decisions must be made, the definitive diagnosis can be provided by a nondecalcified bone biopsy of the iliac crest.

7. The answer is E. Fibrositis, or fibromyalgia, is a major cause of generalized aching and pain, often associated with nonrestorative sleep; the aching typically is exacerbated by cold, damp weather. The cause of fibrositis is unknown, but the sleep disturbance appears to be important. Major differential considerations in the elderly include polymyalgia rheumatica, inflammatory rheumatic syndromes (e.g., rheumatoid arthritis, polymyositis), and endocrinopathies (e.g., hyper- and hypothyroidism, hyperparathyroidism, metabolic bone disease). Fibrositis can be the initial manifestation of a malignancy, especially when bone involvement is present (e.g., multiple myeloma). Depression commonly is associated with fibrositis; fibrositis may be the only clear manifestation of a masked depression. Alzheimer's disease is not associated with fibrositis.

8. The answer is C. The prevalence of asymptomatic calcification of cartilage, or chondrocalcinosis, increases progressively with age and may be seen in as many as 25% of elderly patients, especially in knee joints. Chondrocalcinosis is a typical accompaniment of osteoarthritis, and osteoarthritis is the most common form of clinically symptomatic joint disease associated with calcium pyrophosphate dihydrate (CPPD) deposition. Pseudogout—or liberation of CPPD crystals into joints causing acute inflammation that simulates gout—can occur in apparently normal joints or in joints clinically affected by osteoarthritis. Probably the least common clinical form of CPPD deposition is pseudo-rheumatoid arthritis, a polyarticular joint disease of the joints typically involved in rheumatoid arthritis but usually without systemic features, morning stiffness, or evidence of chronic inflammation. Periarticular inflammation associated with radiographically visible calcium deposits occurs in calcium hydroxyapatite disease, and Milwaukee shoulder is much more commonly caused by these crystals than by CPPD crystals.

9. The answer is D. Extra-articular manifestations are features of highly expressed rheumatoid arthritis, and subcutaneous nodules, eye involvement, hematologic changes, and pulmonary interstitial disease are some of the most common of these expressions. Thrombocytosis and anemia of chronic disease are typical hematologic features; ocular manifestations include sicca complex, scleritis, and episcleritis. Anterior uveitis is a typical manifestation of the spondyloarthropathies, not rheumatoid arthritis. Vasculitis is one of the most serious complications of rheumatoid arthritis and can take several forms; small-vessel ("leukocytoclastic") vasculitis is more common than arteritis involving medium-sized arteries. Finding such extra-articular features in an inflammatory arthritis may be important for diagnosis, therapy, and prognosis.

10. The answer is D. Systemic lupus erythematosus that begins in the geriatric years often presents subtly, with mild skin disease, photosensitivity, pleuritis, or pericarditis. There is no gender predilection, which is in contrast to the female predominance seen in younger lupus patients. The disease also seems to be less severe in the elderly; renal and serious CNS involvement are uncommon, and many patients do not require corticosteroid treatment. Lupus pneumonitis and pulmonary fibrosis are more common in elderly patients than in younger lupus patients.

11. The answer is C. Hydroxyapatite arthropathy is a microcrystalline joint disorder that was first described in the shoulder (Milwaukee shoulder) but also occurs commonly in the knee and less often in the hip or other joints. The characteristic arthropathy involves the formation of large effusions that typically are noninflammatory. Severe destructive joint changes are common, and periarticular tendon dissolution or ruptures often are associated with the arthropathy (e.g., rotator cuff instability in Milwaukee shoulder). Hydroxyapatite crystals also are common in effusions of severe degenerative joint disease, where they may coexist with calcium pyrophosphate dihydrate (CPPD) crystals. Joint fluid that contains calcium hydroxyapatite can be tested using Alizarin red stain. This calcium stain is positive when either hydroxyapatite or CPPD crystals are present. If CPPD crystals are not seen on polarized light microscopy, positive staining typically is due to hydroxyapatite arthropathy. The actual crystal is visible only on electron microscopy.

12. The answer is C. The symptom complex described is a classic case of trochanteric bursitis. Physical examination of a patient with trochanteric bursitis reveals extreme tenderness on palpation over the affected bursa, at the superior and lateral aspect of the greater trochanter. The FABER maneuver (flexion, abduction, and external rotation of the hip) often reproduces pain as does adduction across the midline. Most cases occur in the elderly, and predisposing causes are unknown. Most patients require instillation of a long-acting corticosteroid and local anesthetic combination into the bursa for relief.

Both osteoarthritis and avascular necrosis of the hip hurt most prominently in the groin. Pain from osteoarthritis comes on gradually with activity; pain from avascular necrosis more often is sudden in onset and hurts even at rest. Meralgia paresthetica is a sensation of numbness or impaired sensation felt in the anterolateral thigh due to compression of the lateral femoral cutaneous nerve; it usually does not present solely as pain. Sciatica can radiate down the leg but typically is more lateral and posterior. It typically is associated with back pain, an electric-shock sensation traveling to the foot, and neurologic abnormalities of the ipsilateral leg.

13. The answer is D. Inflammatory synovitis in rheumatoid arthritis that does not respond to nonsteroidal anti-inflammatory agents and conservative measures in the first few months of illness usually requires disease-modifying treatment. Certainly, active inflammatory joint disease that is present for longer than 1 year is unlikely to remit spontaneously and typically requires long-term treatment with a drug such as gold. Progressive deformities and radiographic evidence of erosive joint disease suggest more advanced, destructive disease and are even more compelling reasons to begin treatment with a disease-modifying drug. Chronic joint pain in rheumatoid arthritis can be caused by factors other than inflammatory synovitis (e.g., degenerative joint disease secondary to previous inflammation). This consideration is especially important in elderly patients with disease of long duration; joints severely affected by secondary degenerative change will not show therapeutic response to treatment with a disease-modifying agent.

14. The answer is A. Isolated intracranial vasculitis (also referred to as isolated, or granulomatous, angiitis of the CNS) is a disorder that is histologically similar to giant cell arteritis and that predominantly affects small arteries and veins of the CNS, although any size vessel can be affected. The disease is limited to the brain and spinal cord.

Clinically, most patients experience persistent, severe headache and exhibit signs of an altered mental status; confusion, dementia, and depression or other psychological manifestations are common. Focal neurologic defects become more common as the disease progresses, and as many as 80% of patients with established disease have multifocal deficits of neurologic function.

Because the disease is confined to the CNS, constitutional complaints (e.g., fever, malaise) and other organ system involvement are uncommon. Therefore, myalgias, arthralgias, and mild peripheral neuropathy would not occur more frequently than they do in the general elderly population. Funduscopic findings of microaneurysms and hemorrhage are suggestive of diabetes mellitus and are not features of isolated intracranial vasculitis.

Likewise, laboratory findings usually are normal and not helpful in securing the diagnosis. Most often, the erythrocyte sedimentation rate is normal, and rheumatoid factor and antinuclear antibody are not elevated; regardless, rheumatoid factor and antinuclear antibody elevation do not suggest the presence of isolated intracranial vasculitis.

Brain arteriography or leptomeningeal biopsy is required for the diagnosis; a high degree of suspicion should be present before attempting these procedures. In the classic case, arteriography reveals beading or segmental narrowing of multiple small arteries rather than the proximal carotid artery disease that is more typical of atherosclerosis. Treatment with cytotoxic agents and corticosteroids can significantly improve the prognosis for patients with this otherwise fatal disease.

15. The answer is A. Pes anserine bursitis is the most likely cause of this woman's complaints, as strongly suggested by the pain she experiences when her knees are pressed together. The pes anserine bursa lies about 2 inches below the medial joint line, underneath the conjoined tendons of the sartorius, gracilis, and semitendinous muscles. Palpation over this bursa causes pain when it is inflamed, hence the nocturnal symptoms this patient describes. The setting is a typical one (i.e., an elderly woman with physical findings of degenerative arthritis of the knee and varus deformity). Instillation of a long-acting corticosteroid typically is required for long-term relief. The nocturnal pain and tenderness are not typical for medial compartment degenerative joint disease. Avascular necrosis of the medial tibial plateau may be seen in some elderly patients, usually after relatively minor trauma, but it typically is associated with sudden severe pain both at rest and with ambulation. Popliteal, or Baker's, cysts are synovial fluid–filled sacs that are felt in the popliteal space and not medially; they usually are not painful.

16. The answer is D. Erosive arthritis is a feature of rheumatoid arthritis and, as such, would suggest that Sjögren's syndrome is secondary to rheumatoid arthritis and, thus, is not a primary disorder. Sjögren's syndrome is an autoimmune exocrinopathy involving lymphocytic infiltration of lacrimal and salivary glands, which characteristically presents as dry mouth (xerostomia), dry eyes (keratoconjunctivitis sicca), and variable salivary gland enlargement. Sjögren's syndrome can occur as a primary disorder (i.e., alone, or with characteristic organ involvement and more widespread exocrine gland dysfunction) or as a secondary disorder (i.e., with features usually limited to lacrimal and salivary gland abnormalities in the setting of another rheumatic disease such as rheumatoid arthritis or systemic lupus erythematosus). Different HLA associations (i.e., HLA-DR3 in the primary form and HLA-DR4 in the secondary form) suggest that these are distinct entities. Sjögren's syndrome is quite common in the elderly, in whom it often manifests as isolated lacrimal and salivary gland complaints. Xerostomia in these patients must be distinguished from that caused by commonly administered drugs (e.g., tricyclic antidepressants, phenothiazines). Peripheral neuropathies can be seen in primary Sjögren's syndrome as well as in several of the rheumatoid diseases that can be associated with Sjögren's syndrome.

17. The answer is E. The American Society of Anesthesiologists has adopted the Dripps Physical Status Scale, which is useful in stratifying the risk factors for death in elderly patients being considered for surgery. The factors considered include any underlying disorders as well as the reason for the surgery. Class I patients are at the lowest risk due to the absence of any significant diseases. Class II patients have mild to moderate systemic disease, and class III patients have severe disease. Classes IV and V include patients with life-threatening disorders and those who are dying. Patients who are over the age of 80 are placed in class II even if they have no evident disease because of diminished physiologic reserve and a greater prevalence of covert cardiopulmonary disease. Those who are malnourished are thought to be at a greater risk for serious infection and poor wound healing (a serum albumin of 2.7 g/dl reflects malnutrition). Cardiovascular disorders (e.g., unstable angina, conduction disturbances, arrhythmias, congestive heart failure) are the most significant risk factors for surgical mortality in the elderly. Myocardial infarction within the last 6 months is especially important in increasing the risk of death. Postoperative pulmonary complications (e.g., hypoventilation, atelectasis, pneumonia, inability to be weaned from a ventilator) are significantly more common in patients who have COPD. Obesity also can increase the risk of hypoventilation and pneumonia. Hypertension by itself is not a risk unless associated with end-organ failure.

18. The answer is C. Prosthetic knee replacement is unlikely to result in improved mobility in a patient with joint ankylosis because of muscle contracture around the joint. Patients with rheumatoid arthritis, however, undergo successful total knee replacement as often as those with osteoarthritis, and varus or valgus deformities also can be corrected by the surgery with a good outcome. Radiography may underestimate the severity of clinical disease; therefore, total joint replacement should not be postponed on the basis of only moderate radiographic change. Although a history of thrombophlebitis would warrant extra pre- and postoperative care as well as the use of prophylactic anticoagulation regimens or intermittent leg compression, thrombophlebitis would not necessarily be a contraindication to the surgery.

19. The answer is B. Auranofin is an analogue of gold thioglucose that can be administered orally. Although it may be less effective than injectable gold for the treatment of arthritis, it is less toxic than the intramuscular preparation. Diarrhea is a common side effect but it often is self-limited and rarely requires discontinuation of therapy. Cutaneous reactions, mucosal lesions, eosinophilia, and proteinuria are other common side effects.

20. The answer is B. Amyloidosis is a term used to describe several disorders, all of which are characterized by accumulation of insoluble proteins (amyloid fibrils) in various organs. In primary amyloidosis (often associated with multiple myeloma), immunoglobulin light chains accumulate in the tongue, skin, cardiac and skeletal muscle, peripheral nerves, and visceral organs, causing dysfunction. Secondary amyloidosis develops in patients with chronic inflammatory diseases (e.g., rheumatoid arthritis) and is characterized by tissue accumulation of an insoluble protein derived from serum amyloid A; visceral organ involvement is most typical, and nephrotic syndrome is a classic presentation. Both primary and secondary amyloidosis are more common in the elderly due to the fact that it takes years for the tissue deposition to cause organ dysfunction.

Senile amyloidosis refers to a form of amyloidosis that only occurs in the elderly, in which heart and brain involvement are common but kidney involvement is not. The protein responsible for senile amyloidosis has not been characterized, but it apparently is not an immunoglobulin fragment and probably is different from that found in secondary amyloidosis. Most often, symptoms do not develop and myocardial function is preserved in senile amyloidosis, even with extensive infiltration; death due to arrhythmia would be unlikely in a patient with this disorder. The diagnosis of primary and secondary amyloidosis usually is made by skin or rectal biopsy, although biopsy of an involved organ will show the deposits. The diagnosis of senile amyloidosis usually is made at autopsy.

21. The answer is B. Cancer occurs in 10%–25% of patients with polymyositis or dermatomyositis. Although some studies have suggested that dermatomyositis is more commonly associated with malignancy than is polymyositis, most studies show an equal risk. The malignancies typically found in the elderly population are the ones that are most commonly associated with polymyositis or dermatomyositis (i.e., lung, gastrointestinal, breast, and genitourinary cancers). Screening history, physical examination, and routine laboratory testing are indicated in the search for a malignancy; abnormal findings should be followed carefully with more detailed and specific testing when cancer is suspected in an elderly patient. Removal of a malignancy may result in improvement or remission of the polymyositis, but cure is rare. These patients typically require corticosteroids or other immunomodulatory medication. Vasculitis is a common association only in juvenile dermatomyositis.

22. The answer is A. Polymyalgia rheumatica is a disease that is rare before the age of 50 but is increasingly more common in succeeding decades, affecting as many as 5 in 1000 persons in the geriatric age-group. The disease is characterized by a gradual or acute onset of aching and stiffness in the proximal hip and shoulder girdles, usually accompanied by constitutional complaints. Prominent fatigue, low-grade fever, malaise, and weight loss are common. Although muscle aching is a prominent feature and mild proximal muscle tenderness may occur, muscle weakness is not a feature of this disease. A synovitis has been described and may underlie the proximal muscle aching; radionuclide bone scanning often shows proximal joint uptake, and mildly inflammatory knee synovitis has been described. Laboratory abnormalities are nonspecific and represent those of a chronic inflammatory state; the erythrocyte sedimentation rate is markedly elevated in 99% of cases and usually should be abnormal before the diagnosis is considered. Associated abnormalities may include normocytic, normochromic anemia, increased α_2 globulin levels, and mildly abnormal liver function testing (e.g., elevated serum alkaline phosphatase level).

Polymyalgia rheumatica is a disease of exclusion, and the differential diagnosis always includes rheumatoid arthritis, polymyositis, endocrine disorders, and malignancies. When the diagnosis of polymyalgia rheumatica is made, there should be a careful search for evidence of giant cell (temporal) arteritis, as the diseases are closely associated.

23–26. The answers are: 23-F, 24-T, 25-F, 26-T. Both allopurinol and probenecid decrease the serum level of uric acid—allopurinol by decreasing uric acid production and probenecid by increasing renal excretion of uric acid. In patients with gout, tissue deposition of urate can be reversed by employing such drugs, if a serum uric acid level below 7 mg/dl can be maintained. At such levels, the serum no longer is saturated with uric acid and tissue deposits can be mobilized. Colchicine and indomethacin affect only the inflammatory response excited by the uric acid crystals and have no effect on serum uric acid level or tissue deposition of urate.

27–30. The answers are: 27-F, 28-T, 29-T, 30-F. The lowering of serum uric acid levels is undertaken to prevent or treat the complications of chronic urate deposition in tissues, most commonly acute, recurrent, or tophaceous gout. In the elderly, the risks and inconvenience of chronic drug treatment must be weighed against the potential benefits of preventing acute attacks of gout and reducing tophaceous deposits in soft tissue and joints. The benefits may not outweigh the risks in someone who has only a few years to live and whose functional status is unlikely to be improved by the decision to treat. In some patients, treatment of acute attacks may be sufficient therapy.

However, when an elderly patient is otherwise healthy and able to tolerate the potential risk of a drug reaction, chronic urate reduction therapy with allopurinol or uricosuric agents may be useful in preventing recurrent attacks of acute gout and in solubilizing tophaceous deposits. Renal function impairment rarely is due to urate deposition and is not an indication for treatment. Urolithiasis itself is not an indication for treatment, although a patient with a history of uric acid stones might be treated with allopurinol. Some physicians might even treat calcium stones when urate acts as a nidus for stone formation.

31–34. The answers are: 31-T, 32-T, 33-F, 34-F. Vertebral compression fractures are common in the elderly as a result of osteoporosis. Fractures typically occur with the minimal trauma of sneezing or a bumpy car ride. The most common location is the lower thoracic or upper lumbar vertebrae. Severe pain is typical in the acute period and should be treated with bed rest and pain relief medication. Within 1 or 2 weeks, however, ambulation usually can be encouraged. In addition, a lumbar corset may help with pain relief and early mobilization. Truncal casting or bracing usually is poorly tolerated and unnecessary, as is surgical fixation. Neurologic compromise is extremely unusual, and most patients are relatively free of pain within about 3 months.

35–38. The answers are: 35-T, 36-F, 37-T, 38-F. Nonsteroidal anti-inflammatory drugs (NSAIDs) must be used cautiously in elderly patients due to the increased risk for CNS, gastrointestinal, hematologic, and renal toxicity in older patients treated with these drugs.

A specific caveat is never to combine indomethacin with triamterene, since indomethacin blocks the compensatory renal prostaglandin synthesis necessary to avoid triamterene toxicity. Even in normal young patients this drug combination can produce reversible acute renal failure and hyperkalemia. Elderly patients also are at an increased risk for sodium and water retention and, thus, should be observed for congestive heart failure manifestations, edema, and elevated serum potassium and creatinine levels when given NSAIDs.

Although nonacetylated salicylates are the least likely of the NSAIDs to cause any gastrointestinal toxicity, ibuprofen also is relatively nontoxic to the gastrointestinal tract and is less toxic than aspirin. Perhaps because of a longer half-life and a potential for accumulation, an agent such as piroxicam may cause more peptic ulceration in the elderly and, therefore, requires very careful monitoring if used.

When a patient is given anticoagulants, even the use of nonacetylated salicylates presents problems. The salicylate moiety displaces warfarin from plasma proteins and, thus, prolongs the PT in someone on stable anticoagulation. However, these agents are the only NSAIDs that do not affect platelet function and that can be used safely in patients in whom altered platelet function is a concern (e.g., in the perioperative period).

Finally, the nonacetylated salicylates also are the only NSAIDs that are safe to use in patients with the syndrome of asthma, nasal polyps, and aspirin sensitivity. Any agent that inhibits prostaglandin synthesis (ibuprofen included) can cause wheezing in these patients.

39–42. The answers are: 39-F, 40-T, 41-F, 42-T. Hip fracture is a significant cause of morbidity and mortality in the elderly, especially in women. Low bone density and a tendency to fall are the major factors predisposing to hip fractures in this population. Osteoporosis is characterized by an absolute decrease in bone mass, in contrast to demineralization of bone (osteomalacia).

The process of bone loss begins at some point during adulthood after full skeletal maturity has been attained, and it continues with aging, accelerated by such factors as estrogen loss (menopause) in women, cigarette smoking, and alcohol abuse. Failure to develop maximal bone density during the teenage and young adult years (e.g., due to inadequate calcium intake or physical inactivity) and genetic factors (e.g., northern European heritage, small frame) contribute to a greater effect of bone loss, such that fractures may occur with minimal trauma (e.g., a fall) in high-risk geriatric populations.

In terms of specific risks for osteoporosis (and, hence, hip fractures), obese persons are somewhat protected, probably due to increased loading forces to the skeleton and increased peripheral conversion of androgens to estrogens (in adipose tissue in postmenopausal women). Blacks tend to have greater skeletal density than whites, and whites of northern European ancestry in particular have smaller skeletons. Even blacks with osteoporosis have fewer vertebral and hip fractures than whites. Sedentary lifestyle and lower muscle mass are additional risk factors for osteoporosis.

Type I involutional osteoporosis is associated with greater trabecular bone loss, crush fractures of the distal radius, and fractures of the vertebrae. Type II osteoporosis is associated with both cortical and trabecular bone loss, hip fractures, and evidence of higher than normal levels of circulatory PTH.

Finally, any factor that can cause a tendency for falls will increase the risk for hip fractures in an elderly person. Antipsychotic drugs may worsen orthostatic hypotension (which increases the tendency to fall) and cause confusion (which impairs the ability to break a fall). Poor vision or balance problems are other factors.

43–46. The answers are: 43-T, 44-T, 45-T, 46-F. Giant cell (temporal) arteritis is a vasculitis of the cranial vessels, which affects elderly persons. It is characterized by chronic inflammation of the large vessels, often with giant cells; the temporal artery classically is involved. Giant cell arteritis is closely associated with polymyalgia rheumatica, and patients often have features of both illnesses, including marked elevation of the erythrocyte sedimentation rate and nonspecific laboratory findings of chronic inflammation. Bitemporal headache with intermittent shooting pains, jaw claudication, and scalp tenderness are classic features.

The illness has protean manifestations. An elderly patient can present with constitutional complaints and features of dementia or depression. An elderly patient with a sudden onset of headache also must be evaluated for the diagnosis, especially when symptoms occur in the setting of apparent polymyalgia rheumatica. One of the most dread complications of this disorder involves vasculitis of the ophthalmic or posterior ciliary artery. This inflammation sometimes can present as amaurosis fugax (which patients frequently describe as being similar to having a shade pulled down over one eye) or as any number of other visual complaints (e.g., diplopia, excessive tearing, conjunctivitis, scotomata, photophobia). Blindness usually is not a presenting complaint, but any visual disorder suggests the possibility of giant cell arteritis.

The last patient described apparently is suffering from accelerated hypertension, which is not known to be a presentation of giant cell arteritis.

47–50. The answers are: 47-T, 48-T, 49-F, 50-T. Osteoarthritis is a joint disease in which articular cartilage is lost and subchondral bone is remodeled. Radiographic studies have shown that osteoarthritis most commonly is an asymptomatic polyarticular disease; more than 80% of people over the age of 55 have radiographic evidence of osteoarthritis but far fewer complain of symptoms in the involved joints.

Gender and race appear to be factors in determining which joints are likely to be affected by osteoarthritis. White women with a positive family history are at highest risk for primary generalized osteoarthritis; this disorder is less common in white men and quite rare in black men. Knee osteoarthritis seems to be more common in women, but hip degenerative joint disease occurs with equal frequency in men and women.

Physical activity is not likely to predispose to osteoarthritis in the absence of some specific major joint trauma. Repetitive physical activity may have an effect on which joints will be affected by osteoarthritis, but it is not a factor determining whether a person will develop osteoarthritis.

Osteoarthritis commonly is associated with metabolic diseases. Diabetes mellitus, hemochromatosis, acromegaly, hypothyroidism, alkaptonuria, and Wilson's disease are associated with abnormal cartilage metabolism or accelerated aging of cartilage. Thus, normal stresses on abnormal cartilage predispose to osteoarthritis as do abnormal stresses on normal cartilage.

51–54. The answers are: 51-T, 52-F, 53-T, 54-F. The particular joints involved and the presence or absence of inflammatory features help to distinguish between various forms of arthritis. Inflammatory complaints (e.g., redness, swelling) make erosive osteoarthritis a likely diagnosis. This disorder occurs more often in middle-aged or older women, sometimes with autosomal dominant, gender-influenced characteristics. Erosive arthritis generally presents as more inflammatory features than are typical of osteoarthritis. One form of psoriatic arthritis typically affects the distal interphalangeal joints, either alone or in combination with other joint or spondylitic involvement. Nail pitting or dystrophy often accompanies this "classic" form of psoriatic arthritis, and skin disease usually is present when patients have symptoms of arthritis.

Although an atypical presentation of rheumatoid arthritis is a possibility here, it seems less likely given the joint involvement, intermittency of complaints, and absence of systemic features. Rheumatoid arthritis involving the distal interphalangeal joints of the hand presents as more widespread joint inflammation, characteristically with metacarpophalangeal and proximal interphalangeal joint involvement. In addition, it would be typical to see the wrists and other peripheral joints involved in a generally symmetrical fashion.

Ankylosing spondylitis is an unlikely cause of this elderly woman's complaints. This disease occurs most often in young men and predominantly involves the axial skeleton, especially the sacroiliac joints, and less often the appendicular skeleton.

Gout is another potential diagnosis to consider in this elderly patient, if she had presented with acute inflammation of 1 or 2 joints—even a distal interphalangeal joint of the hand. In women, gout occurs almost exclusively after menopause; it is rarely seen in premenopausal women because of the uricosuric effect of estrogen. Elderly women with gout typically have an associated cause of sustained hyperuricemia, most often chronic thiazide diuretic treatment.

8
Genitourinary Disorders

QUESTIONS

Directions: Each question below contains five suggested answers. Choose the **one best** response to each question.

1. Prostatitis is a common cause of urinary tract infections in men. Treatment of chronic bacterial prostatitis is best accomplished with

(A) erythromycin
(B) carbenicillin
(C) ampicillin
(D) trimethoprim-sulfamethoxazole
(E) minocycline

2. What organism is the most common cause of a urinary tract infection in older people?

(A) *Staphylococcus aureus*
(B) *Staphylococcus epidermidis*
(C) *Escherichia coli*
(D) *Proteus mirabilis*
(E) *Pseudomonas aeruginosa*

3. An elderly patient with normal renal function has a serum sodium concentration of 120 mEq/L and does not appear to be dehydrated. This patient most likely has

(A) a total body sodium deficit
(B) dilutional hyponatremia
(C) a contracted blood volume
(D) diabetes insipidus
(E) Cushing's disease

4. An elderly patient with chronic renal failure due to long-standing, severe hypertension is seen because of chest pain. The patient has received hemodialysis twice weekly for the last 2 years. The major problem on dialysis has been recent episodes of hypotension at the beginning of treatment. The chest pain is located over the trapezius muscle and is moderately reduced by assuming the upright position but exacerbated by deep breathing. The most likely cause of this patient's chest pain is

(A) pericarditis
(B) coronary artery disease
(C) diffuse esophageal spasm
(D) pulmonary embolism
(E) costochondritis

5. Factors that commonly contribute to the hyperkalemia seen in elderly patients with mild to moderate renal failure (i.e., a serum creatinine level of 2–3 mg/dl) include all of the following EXCEPT

(A) gastrointestinal bleeding
(B) elevated potassium intake
(C) age-related reduction of GFR
(D) aldosterone excess
(E) nonsteroidal anti-inflammatory drugs

6. A 78-year-old man is seen because of extreme variations in his urine output. Today he is passing large amounts of urine; however, on some days he passes no urine at all. Physical examination reveals a blood pressure of 180/90 mm Hg but otherwise normal findings. Laboratory findings include a BUN level of 120 mg/dl and a serum creatinine level of 4.2 mg/dl. Urinalysis reveals a specific gravity of 1.010, urine that is negative for protein, glucose, ketone bodies, and blood, and an occasional white blood cell per high-power field on microscopic examination. The most likely cause of this patient's renal insufficiency is

(A) obstructive uropathy
(B) acute glomerulonephritis
(C) acute interstitial nephritis
(D) acute tubular necrosis
(E) chronic renal failure

7. A 71-year-old man is seen in the surgical intensive care unit for acute renal failure. The patient had a cholecystectomy, after which there was a persistent drainage from his biliary catheter associated with spiking fevers to 102° F. He has been taking gentamicin (70 mg every 8 hours) and cephalothin (2 g 4 times a day) for the past 10 days. Over the last 4 days, the serum creatinine level has increased at a rate of 1 mg/dl/day, but urine output has been normal. There has been no history of hypotension at any time during this hospitalization. Physical examination shows normal blood pressure and vital signs, laboratory studies show a creatinine level of 7.1 mg/dl and an unremarkable urinalysis, and renal ultrasonography reveals no evidence of obstruction. The most likely cause of this patient's acute renal failure is

(A) inadequate fluid replacement
(B) hepatorenal syndrome
(C) gentamicin nephrotoxicity
(D) acute glomerulonephritis
(E) acute interstitial nephritis

8. In elderly or debilitated nursing home patients, symptoms of incontinence, fever, and mental confusion and signs of vasomotor collapse may be present in which of the following disorders?

(A) Analgesic nephropathy
(B) Urinary tract infection
(C) Interstitial nephritis
(D) Membranous glomerulonephritis
(E) Renal artery stenosis

9. The most common form of nephrotic syndrome seen in adults is

(A) primary membranous glomerulonephritis
(B) lipoid nephrosis
(C) focal glomerulosclerosis
(D) crescentic glomerulonephritis
(E) amyloidosis

10. Patients with chronic renal failure are likely to present with all of the following clinical manifestations EXCEPT

(A) hypercalcemia
(B) an increased incidence of infection
(C) bleeding abnormalities
(D) pruritus
(E) pericarditis

11. A 70-year-old man who has been maintained on chronic peritoneal dialysis for the past year is seen in the emergency room. He has been very careful regarding technique, but over the last 24 hours he has noticed a mild, cramping abdominal pain. No other pertinent history is elicited. He does not note any cloudiness of the dialysis fluid. Physical examination reveals a temperature of 101° F but otherwise normal vital signs. Abdominal examination reveals the presence of a catheter in place with no erythema but mild periumbilical tenderness. Peritoneal fluid analysis reveals a white blood cell count of 900/mm^3 (80% neutrophils). The most appropriate diagnosis is

(A) uremic peritonitis
(B) bacterial peritonitis
(C) tuberculous peritonitis
(D) gastroenteritis
(E) "walled-off" appendiceal abscess

12. Urinary incontinence is a common complaint among the elderly, which is associated with many physiologic effects of aging. Urgency incontinence, the most common type, is the result of

(A) the inability of the distal urethral mechanism to withstand a sudden rise in intra-abdominal pressure
(B) the inability of the distal urethral mechanism to withstand a sudden rise in intravesicular pressure
(C) the inability to reach the toilet in time
(D) an excessive volume of residual urine
(E) chronic urinary tract infections

Directions: The groups of questions below consist of an introductory premise or case data followed by four statements that pertain to the information given. Indicate whether each statement is **true** or **false**.

Questions 13–16

The initial evaluation of an elderly patient with renal calculi should include each of the following laboratory tests.

13. KUB x-ray
14. Serum calcium and phosphate levels
15. Serum alkaline phosphatase determination
16. Urinalysis

Questions 17–20

In an elderly patient with renal disease, an antibiotic that is renally excreted should be administered with caution. The following agents may be administered to a patient whose renal function is severely compromised.

17. Erythromycin
18. Tobramycin
19. Doxycycline
20. Penicillin G

Questions 21–24

The indications for the surgical removal of urinary calculi include each of the following.

21. Infection
22. Obstruction
23. Mild pain
24. Growth of a silent calculus

Questions 25–28

Evaluation of an elderly patient with erectile failure usually requires each of the following basic tests.

25. Determination of serum prolactin level
26. Determination of serum testosterone level
27. Determination of serum HCG
28. Penile blood pressure measurement

Questions 29–32

When evaluating urinary incontinence in an elderly patient, it is necessary to have a complete history that includes the following information.

29. History of enuresis
30. Institutional living
31. Use of tranquilizers
32. Chronic constipation

Questions 33–36

The following conditions are commonly seen in elderly patients with chronic renal failure.

33. Anemia
34. Hypernatremia
35. Metabolic acidosis
36. Hypophosphatemia

Questions 37–40

Renal artery stenosis in the elderly commonly is associated with the following conditions.

37. Fibromuscular dysplasia
38. Uncontrollable hypertension
39. Abdominal bruit
40. Disparity in kidney size

Questions 41–44

A 73-year-old man who recently had prostate surgery develops a urinary tract infection. *Pseudomonas aeruginosa* is cultured. Suitable therapy includes the following agents.

41. Ceftazidime
42. Cephalothin
43. Carbenicillin indanyl
44. Chloramphenicol

Questions 45–48

A 60-year-old man presents with a complaint of gross painless hematuria. The diagnostic work-up of this patient should include the following procedures.

45. Screening for urinary nitrate reduction

46. Intravenous urography

47. Evaluation of clotting parameters

48. Cystoscopy

Questions 49–52

An 81-year-old man with a recent change in mental status is found to have a serum sodium concentration of 119 mmol/L. The serum osmolality is 265 mOsm/kg, and the urine osmolality is 350 mOsm/kg. Urine sodium excretion is 85 mmol/24 hr. The following are possible causes for this syndrome.

49. Pulmonary tuberculosis

50. Demeclocycline treatment

51. Chlorpropamide treatment

52. Sodium depletion

Questions 53–56

The following statements accurately describe the effects of age on the male reproductive system.

53. The most severe degenerative change in the seminiferous tubules is a thickening of the basement membrane

54. The concentration of spermatozoa in semen samples is unaffected by age

55. Sperm motility declines with age

56. Serum testosterone level declines with age

ANSWERS AND EXPLANATIONS

1. The answer is D. Chronic bacterial prostatitis is the most common cause of recurrent urinary tract infection in men. The majority (> 80%) of cases are caused by *Escherichia coli*. The condition may be occult, with low-grade fever, recurrent bacteriuria, and mild back or pelvic pain. However, patients usually are asymptomatic until significant bacteriuria occurs. Symptoms include back, pelvic, perineal, penile, and scrotal pain as well as dysuria, nocturia, urgency, and frequency.

The treatment of chronic bacterial prostatitis is frequently frustrating for the physician because of the difficulty in achieving penetration of the appropriate antibiotic to the site of the infection. The antibiotic chosen must have good lipid solubility for prostatic tissue. Trimethoprim-sulfamethoxazole is the agent of choice. Treatment involves 6 weeks of continuous therapy. If the patient does not respond to trimethoprim-sulfamethoxazole, erythromycin, carbenicillin, ampicillin, or minocycline can be tried. Newer antimicrobial agents, the quinolones (e.g., norfloxacin, ciprofloxacin), have excellent prostatic penetration and will be particularly effective in resistant or recurrent cases.

2. The answer is C. *Escherichia coli* is responsible for the majority of urinary infections, both initial and recurrent. Other organisms cause infections in patients previously treated with antibiotics or those with complicating factors such as anatomic abnormalities. Species of *Proteus*, *Enterobacter*, *Pseudomonas*, and *Klebsiella* as well as *Staphylococcus aureus* and anaerobes are present in the urine of older people more often than in that of younger people and may cause infection. Prevention of urinary tract infections in the elderly involves maintaining activity and avoiding the use of catheters. Bedridden patients have an increased incidence of urinary tract infections, and fecal incontinence increases the risk of infection in women. Catheters and urinary stones also are associated with a particularly high frequency. When a catheter is used, the best prophylaxis is closed drainage. Complications of active urinary tract infections in the elderly include disorientation and systemic sepsis as well as more typical urinary tract complaints.

3. The answer is B. If a patient with hyponatremia does not show signs of dehydration, then it is likely that he or she is overhydrated, resulting in dilutional hyponatremia. In this state, the blood volume is overexpanded, and the total body sodium is normal. Older patients can become dehydrated and hyponatremic in association with surgery or acute febrile illness. Diabetes insipidus produces hypernatremia and dehydration. Cushing's disease is not a cause of hyponatremia.

4. The answer is A. Chronic renal failure is more common with increasing age, and elderly patients are more often managed with chronic dialysis than renal transplantation. The chest pain experienced by this patient is typical of pericarditis and inflammation of the pericardium, which are common complications in chronic renal failure patients on hemodialysis. These patients also may have inflammation in various serosal linings, including the peritoneum, the pleura, and various joint spaces; the mechanism of this complication is unknown. Although coronary artery disease is common in dialysis patients, the characteristics of the pain in this patient suggest that this is not the diagnosis. Esophageal disease also is common in dialysis patients and should be excluded as a possible cause. In addition, chest wall pain due to various causes is seen frequently in dialysis patients, as it is in the general population. The dialysis-related hypotensive episodes in this patient may be due to increased pericardial fluid pressure restricting cardiac filling (pericardial tamponade), so treatment of the pericarditis may be relatively urgent.

5. The answer is D. Hyperkalemia is defined as a serum potassium concentration greater than 5.5 mEq/L. In mild renal failure, the intrinsic capacity of the kidney to secrete potassium is still adequate. Serum potassium levels vary, but they tend to be higher than normal if intake is not restricted; therefore, exogenous sources of potassium probably should be eliminated. Decreases (not increases) in GFR, aldosterone, and renin add to an elderly person's risk for developing hyperkalemia. Nonsteroidal anti-inflammatory drugs impair GFR in elderly patients who require compensatory renal prostaglandin synthesis for maintenance of normal function. Old age, congestive heart failure, cirrhosis, nephrosis, and diuretic therapy all are situations in which renal prostaglandin synthesis is required. Gastrointestinal bleeding—due to gastritis, ulcer, or malignancy— is a major source of potassium (due to gut uptake from fragmented red blood cells). Renal failure is associated with a higher incidence of gastrointestinal bleeding.

6. The answer is A. The incidence of prostatism in elderly men is so great that it must be considered the primary cause of renal insufficiency until proven otherwise. This patient's history is classic in that he had 1 or 2 days on which he seemed to pass no urine followed by days of high urine flow, a pattern that is caused by the gradual accumulation of large amounts of urine in the collecting system under pressure, which eventually may overcome some degree of obstruction. The high pressure is transmitted back to the kidney and results in renal insufficiency. Acute glomerulonephritis and acute interstitial nephritis are ruled out by the normal results of urinalysis. The possibility of acute tubular necrosis should be considered, but there is no information in the history that suggests recent surgery or nephrotoxic drug intake that would have produced such a problem. With chronic renal failure, a BUN-to-serum creatinine ratio of 10:1 would be more typical. This patient's ratio of 30:1 suggests some degree of prerenal azotemia or a postrenal cause of renal insufficiency (e.g., obstruction). The best screening tool for obstructive uropathy is renal ultrasonography, which would demonstrate hydronephrosis.

7. The answer is C. Approximately 5%–10% of patients treated with gentamicin develop a reversible nonoliguric form of acute renal failure. Although this patient has received standard doses of gentamicin, its accumulation in the kidney has led to increasing renal tubule toxicity. Excretion of gentamicin is decreased in this situation, so gentamicin levels rise and the renal function worsens—a vicious cycle. Nonoliguric renal failure is a typical manifestation of gentamicin nephrotoxicity. Cephalothin is being given to this patient, and its concomitant use potentiates the renal toxicity of gentamicin. Although the patient could have obstructive uropathy, the negative results of ultrasonography strongly indicate otherwise. Cephalothin can produce an acute interstitial nephritis, but the patient's clinical course is much more compatible with gentamicin nephrotoxicity. Acute glomerulonephritis usually is associated with hypertension and an active urinary sediment containing casts, protein, and red blood cells. Both dehydration (with inadequate fluid replacement) and hepatorenal syndrome would be associated with decreased urine output in the absence of renal dysfunction.

8. The answer is B. An elderly or debilitated nursing home patient with a urinary tract infection such as cystitis may not present with the typical symptoms of dysuria, frequency, and urgency seen in the younger patient but may present primarily with incontinence, fever, chills, mental confusion, or signs of vasomotor instability. In the geriatric patient, urinary tract infection often occurs in the presence of renal calculi, prostatic hyperplasia, or hypotonic bladder with residual urine and can initially present as a gram-negative bacteremia or septicemia. Elderly patients presenting with signs and symptoms suggesting gram-negative bacteremia and vasomotor collapse require vigorous hospitalized care, with broad-spectrum antibiotics and intravenous fluids to support blood pressure.

9. The answer is A. Features of nephrotic syndrome (i.e., albuminuria, hypoalbuminemia, hyperlipidemia, edema) result from excessive leakage of plasma proteins through the glomerular capillary wall into the urine. Immunologic, metabolic, vascular, and biochemical disorders and toxic injuries all can lead to this clinical picture by injury to the glomeruli; injury to the renal tubule or interstitium does not lead to nephrotic syndrome.

Membranous nephropathy is the most common form of primary glomerular disease in adults (in contrast to minimal lesion, or minimal change disease, in children). It also is a secondary feature of drug reactions (e.g., gold, penicillamine, captopril) and systemic diseases that can occur in the elderly (e.g., chronic hepatitis B antigenemia, neoplasia, Sjögren's syndrome, systemic lupus erythematosus).

Focal glomerulosclerosis is seen in about 5%–12% of renal biopsies in adult patients with nephrotic syndrome. Crescentic glomerulonephritis and amyloidosis are uncommon causes, but amyloidosis may appear more commonly in chronic inflammatory diseases such as rheumatoid arthritis.

10. The answer is A. Patients with chronic renal failure typically are hypocalcemic as a result of hyperphosphatemia as well as impaired vitamin D activity. Infections are more common in uremic patients, due to impaired cell-mediated immunity and decreased neutrophil chemotaxis. An increased tendency to bleeding in chronic renal failure patients is the result of defects in platelet adhesion and aggregation, which can be corrected somewhat by dialysis. Pruritus often occurs for unknown reasons. Pericarditis is a common feature of end-stage renal disease, and it is controlled best with adequate dialysis. Other common uremic abnormalities include accelerated atherosclerosis; anemia; electrolyte disorders; anorexia, nausea, and vomiting; renal osteodystrophy; and neuromyopathies.

Renal disease in older people often is secondary to other diseases, and once the diagnosis of chronic renal failure is made, the cause should be identified. The presenting signs of chronic renal failure in the elderly differ from those in younger patients in several ways. Substantially higher serum creatinine levels occur in younger patients than in older people. The serum creatinine level in older people does not indicate the extent of renal failure, and so diagnosis may be delayed. Hypertension, worsening of preexisting heart failure, or gastrointestinal bleeding may appear before uremic manifestations.

11. The answer is B. The most likely cause of this clinical picture is acute bacterial peritonitis. This complication occurs in 10%–20% of renal patients maintained on chronic ambulatory peritoneal dialysis. The typical organisms are *Staphylococcus aureus* and *Staphylococcus epidermidis*. Peritonitis may become a recurrent problem in patients on chronic ambulatory peritoneal dialysis and may be due to contamination of the peritoneal catheter or the presence of an intra-abdominal abscess. Initial antibiotic coverage should include an antistaphylococcal agent. Although uremic peritonitis does occur in dialysis patients as do a variety of intra-abdominal disorders (e.g., gastroenteritis, tuberculous peritonitis, perforated viscus), in this clinical setting the physician must first treat bacterial peritonitis while considering these less likely entities.

12. The answer is B. The most common type of incontinence in the elderly is called "urgency" incontinence, accounting for approximately 60% of cases. It is the result of uninhibited detrusor contractions that are not coordinated with urethral sphincter opening, and it causes urgency, frequency, and small volume voiding. Stress incontinence (childbirth incontinence), a less common problem occurring in elderly women, results from the inability of the distal urethral mechanism to adjust to sudden increases in intra-abdominal pressure such as occur with coughing. Overflow incontinence results from excessive residual volume and may present as a persistent daytime dribble. It can be due to anatomic obstruction of outflow (e.g., prostatism) or neuropathic impairment of detrusor contraction. Functional incontinence is the inability to reach the toilet in time. It is due to psychological factors, impaired mobility, rigid institutional schedules, and inconvenient location of the toilet. Iatrogenic incontinence is caused by diuretic, anticholinergic, or sedative drugs and can worsen any of the other causes of incontinence.

13–16. The answers are: 13-T, 14-T, 15-T, 16-T. Renal calculi in the aged can cause acute or chronic renal disease and lead to renal insufficiency. The patient who presents with the characteristic signs and symptoms of a urinary tract calculus generally requires minimum laboratory tests during initial evaluation. A plain abdominal and pelvic radiograph (KUB x-ray) identifies stones in 90% of the cases. An IVP may be required to demonstrate small stones, radiolucent stones such as uric acid stones, and the anatomic site of the stone within the urinary tract.

Serum calcium, phosphate, and alkaline phosphatase levels are important to identify hypercalcemic states, such as sarcoidosis, and hyperparathyroidism with metabolic bone diseases. A urinalysis is important to identify infection, particularly infection with urea-splitting organisms and their association with triple phosphate stones, a cause of infection that is more common in the elderly.

Evaluation beyond the initial stage frequently includes serum PTH level and 24-hour urine collection for measurement of total calcium and uric acid excretion. When the stone is passed it should be analyzed for its mineral composition.

Immobilization for longer than 2 weeks due to paralysis or a fracture requiring a body cast may lead to hypercalciuria (urinary calcium excretion exceeding 500 mg/day), which leads to calcium stone formation. This reaction to immobilization is increased in the aged.

17–20. The answers are: 17-T, 18-F, 19-T, 20-F. When renal function is severely compromised, drugs cannot be excreted by the kidney. The lack of renal excretion of a particular drug or its metabolites must be considered before treatment is undertaken.

Penicillin G and tobramycin are antibiotics that are renally excreted. In the renally compromised patient, penicillins can cause allergic interstitial nephritis. Seizures and platelet dysfunction can occur at high blood levels of penicillin in the presence of renal disease, and hyperkalemia can occur due to the inability of the kidney to excrete the extra potassium load. Tobramycin causes nephrotoxicity and ototoxicity, and peak-and-trough blood levels of tobramycin are the best guide to therapy. Penicillin administered concurrently with tobramycin may cause subtherapeutic blood levels.

Both erythromycin and doxycycline are excreted in the bile and feces; thus, they are useful in the treatment of infections in patients with renal insufficiency, although erythromycin may be ototoxic in renal failure. Doxycycline is the tetracycline of choice for the treatment of extrarenal infections in the presence of renal disease; however, it may potentiate acidosis and raise serum phosphorus levels and BUN.

21–24. The answers are: 21-T, 22-T, 23-F, 24-T. Any obvious obstruction in an elderly person must be remedied, although general anesthesia is somewhat riskier in the elderly than in the young. The indications for the surgical removal of urinary calculi include infection, obstruction, severe pain, and growth of a silent calculus. When infection is present proximal to a calculus, antibiotic therapy should be instituted to control the infection and removal of the calculus should be delayed. A calculus should be removed if it is causing severe obstruction with potential renal damage. Temporary relief may be obtained by ureteral catheter drainage of urine. Mild pain from a urinary calculus can be controlled with analgesics. More severe pain that cannot be controlled satisfactorily is a major indication for removal of the calculus. Growth of a silent calculus during observation also is an indication for removal. Calculi can be monitored without specific treatment if they remain asymptomatic.

25–28. The answers are: 25-T, 26-T, 27-F, 28-T. Delay in obtaining an erection is a normal physiologic phenomenon in elderly men. However, sexual dysfunction in the elderly man generally presents as loss of libido or erectile failure. Psychogenic causes are common; depression is an especially frequent and important cause of impotence in elderly men.

If the history and physical examination do not reveal an obvious cause of an impotence problem that has been present for several months, serum testosterone and prolactin levels should be evaluated. Serum FSH and LH levels also should be checked if the testosterone level is low to identify a pituitary cause since hormone manipulation therapy for testicular or pituitary problems often restores potency. Bromocriptine treatment for hyperprolactinemia also is effective, whether or not a pituitary adenoma can be found. HCG levels are not helpful in the routine evaluation of impotence.

Penile blood pressure determinations, if available, may indicate inadequate penile blood flow. When this is related to obstruction of major pelvic vessels, revascularization procedures can be used. Because revascularization of small vessels has not been particularly successful, treatment by implantation of a prosthesis may be indicated.

29–32. The answers are: 29-T, 30-T, 31-T, 32-T. Urinary incontinence in the elderly often is multifactorial. Generally, as age increases, it is more likely that the condition is caused by neurologic factors. Because the etiology frequently is complex, a detailed history is perhaps the most important part of the diagnostic evaluation.

It is important to obtain a history of continence. The age that continence is attained, a history of enuresis, a family history of incontinence, and a history of a "weak bladder" are important components of the patient history. It should be determined if the degree of continence is personally and socially acceptable. In institutions, emphasis placed on the use of bedpans rather than commodes, lack of privacy, and confusion caused by unmarked lavatories all are factors that can foster incontinence.

A medication history should be obtained to identify drug-related causes of incontinence (e.g., use of diuretics, anticholinergics, antidepressants, antipsychotics, or hypnotics). The setting in which incontinence occurs also is important: Urgency and frequent small-volume voidings suggest detrusor instability (urgency incontinence), and constant dribbling suggests overflow incontinence. Also, patients with gait disturbances or arthritis may have functional incontinence— they cannot get to the toilet in time. Multiparous women with prolapsed urethrae have sphincteric (stress) incontinence and often lose bladder control with coughing or laughing. Finally, constipation severe enough to cause impaction can result in overflow incontinence by bladder outlet obstruction.

33–36. The answers are: 33-T, 34-F, 35-T, 36-F. Normochromic, normocytic anemia is commonly seen in patients with chronic renal failure. The anemia is partly caused by the decreased production and survival time of red blood cells, but it can be substantially corrected by giving erythropoietin. Hypernatremia is uncommon in chronic renal failure patients, although it has been encountered in patients on peritoneal dialysis when high glucose concentrations are added to the dialysate. The osmoreceptor mechanism is operating; therefore, serum sodium levels are normal. Elderly patients sometimes have dilutional hyponatremia as a result of dialysis-related salt and water fluxes. Progressive renal failure causes metabolic acidosis. As the disease advances, total daily excretion of acid drops below the concentrations necessary for maintenance of the external balance of hydrogen ions. Decreasing ability of the kidney to excrete phosphates can produce hyperphosphatemia. Serum phosphate levels begin to rise when the GFR falls below about 25% of normal.

37–40. The answers are: 37-F, 38-T, 39-T, 40-T. Renal artery stenosis is due to fibromuscular dysplasia of arterial tissue or to atherosclerosis. Fibromuscular dysplasia occurs mainly in women who are between 20 and 30 years old; atherosclerosis of the renal arteries is the primary cause in patients older than 45 with signs of diffuse atherosclerosis. The hypertension related to renal artery stenosis must be differentiated from essential hypertension: Suspicion is confirmed by a history of recent, rapid onset of the hypertension, by difficulty in controlling blood pressure with antihypertensive medication, and by the presence of flank bruits. Other criteria for screening for renal artery stenosis in older people include an age greater than 45 years at the onset of hypertension and eligibility for surgical intervention. Digital subtraction angiography, radioisotope scanning, and rapid-sequence intravenous urography all can be useful in the further evaluation of a patient who is likely to have this disorder. A significant finding on ultrasonography or IVP is a disparity in kidney size: A difference of about 2 cm is suggestive of unilateral renal artery stenosis.

41–44. The answers are: 41-T, 42-F, 43-T, 44-F. Ceftazidime, a third-generation cephalosporin, has greater activity against *Pseudomonas* infections than the other third-generation cephalosporins. Carbenicillin is less effective against *Pseudomonas* than other antipseudomonas penicillins (e.g., azlocillin); however, carbenicillin indanyl accumulates in the urine and, therefore, is useful for treatment of urinary tract *Pseudomonas* infections. Imipenem is useful for serious hospital-acquired *Pseudomonas* infections; however, organisms may become resistant during therapy. Gentamicin and other aminoglycosides also are effective against *Pseudomonas*, but they are used chiefly for life-threatening infections because of their toxicity. Chloramphenicol and the first-generation cephalosporins such as cephalothin are not effective against *Pseudomonas*.

45–48. The answers are: 45-F, 46-T, 47-T, 48-T. Patients with gross painless hematuria must be evaluated for a urinary tract neoplasm. The majority of patients with urothelial neoplasms or renal parenchymal tumors experience hematuria, and it is the single presenting complaint of most patients, regardless of the involved level of the urinary tract. However, absence of hematuria does not rule out a urologic tumor. Bladder trabeculation and diverticular formation are common in elderly men due to prostate-related outlet obstruction from prostatism, and there is an increased incidence of bladder tumors found in these diverticuli.

Evaluation of clotting parameters should be done in any patient who presents with bleeding. Intravenous urography and cystoscopy should be performed in a patient with hematuria unless the source of bleeding is certain. Nitrate reduction testing is useful only when screening for infections.

49–52. The answers are: 49-T, 50-F, 51-T, 52-F. The syndrome of inappropriate secretion of ADH (SIADH) occurs when ADH is produced without a physiologic cause. It manifests as hyponatremia and inappropriate urinary sodium loss without volume contraction. As urinary sodium excretion increases, the serum sodium concentration decreases. Blood volume is maintained due to water retention. Pulmonary disorders such as tuberculosis cause SIADH through unknown mechanisms. Chlorpropamide, a hypoglycemic agent used in the treatment of diabetes mellitus, can cause SIADH. The drug causes the kidney to be responsive to levels of ADH that normally are too low to stimulate renal reabsorption of water. Demeclocycline, on the other hand, blocks the action of ADH and may be used in the treatment of SIADH. When hyponatremia results from sodium depletion (e.g., volume depletion states), rather than ADH excess, renal homeostatic mechanisms retain sodium, and urinary sodium excretion is low, usually less than 20 mmol/24 hr.

53–56. The answers are: 53-T, 54-F, 55-T, 56-T. A number of age-related degenerative changes in the histologic appearance of the seminiferous tubules have been reported. The most important of these is a thickening of the basement membrane resulting from peritubular collagen deposition. Spermatozoa content of semen declines with age, as evidenced by the fact that men in their 60s typically produce semen samples consisting of 70% spermatozoa, whereas samples from men in their 80s contain only about 50%. Sperm motility has been reported to decrease somewhat with age; however, decreased motility has also been associated with the longer interejaculatory interval typical of elderly men. Numerous studies have reported reduction of serum testosterone levels. The decline seems to begin at about age 50 and continue into the 80s and 90s. The range of testosterone concentration among elderly men is so wide, however, that many of these people have values well above normal.

9 Endocrine and Metabolic Disorders

QUESTIONS

Directions: Each question below contains five suggested answers. Choose the **one best** response to each question.

1. Primary hyperparathyroidism is detected with increasing frequency in adults over age 50. Most patients are asymptomatic, with a high serum calcium level. When symptoms are present, they often are varied and vague. All of the following manifestations of primary hyperparathyroidism are caused by hypercalcemia EXCEPT

(A) polyuria
(B) hypertension
(C) bone pain
(D) memory impairment
(E) proximal muscle weakness

2. The incidence of neuropathic complications of diabetes increases with the duration of the disease. An elderly diabetic patient who has autonomic neuropathy may present with all of the following complications EXCEPT

(A) bradycardia
(B) impotence
(C) urinary retention
(D) nocturnal diarrhea
(E) decreased awareness of hypoglycemia

3. Hyponatremia in the elderly is most likely to be associated with which of the following conditions?

(A) Diabetes insipidus
(B) Diabetic ketoacidosis
(C) Coma
(D) Bronchogenic carcinoma
(E) Mannitol administration

4. A 68-year-old woman complains of cold intolerance, chronic sleepiness, and weight gain despite a decreased appetite. Physical examination reveals facial and peripheral edema and a slight hearing impairment. Hypothyroidism is suspected. Which of the following laboratory values would confirm a thyroid cause of this patient's hypothyroidism?

(A) A low free T_4 index with a low serum T_3 level
(B) A low free T_4 index with a low serum TSH level
(C) A low free T_4 index with a high serum TSH level
(D) A high free T_4 index with a low serum TSH level
(E) Low thyroid antibody levels

5. Endocrine disorders should not be overlooked in the search for a cause of impotence. Which of the following hormone alterations is most indicative of a primary testicular cause of impotence?

(A) Decreased testosterone level
(B) Increased prolactin level
(C) Increased LH level
(D) Increased estrogen level
(E) Increased thyroid hormone level

6. Hypercalcemia in elderly patients may be due to all of the following nonparathyroid causes EXCEPT

(A) bronchogenic carcinoma
(B) multiple myeloma
(C) hyperthyroidism
(D) loop diuretics
(E) antacids

7. A 64-year-old man with mild type II diabetes frequently stays in hotels because his job involves traveling. He has trouble maintaining a suitable diet with restaurant meals and refuses to consider the use of insulin injections. All of the following agents could be tried in this patient EXCEPT

(A) acetohexamide
(B) chlorpropamide
(C) glyburide
(D) sulfanilamide
(E) tolbutamide

8. Osteoporosis is a common disease in the elderly and the major factor underlying hip fractures that frequently occur in this age-group. Elderly women are the most frequently affected. Major risk factors for osteoporosis in this population include all of the following EXCEPT

(A) early menopause
(B) obesity
(C) short stature
(D) cigarette smoking
(E) sedentary lifestyle

9. A 65-year-old woman complains of listlessness, heat intolerance, and a 20-lb weight loss. Physical examination reveals a depressed appearing woman with an irregularly irregular pulse rate of 120/min but no evidence of goiter or thyroid nodules. Atrial fibrillation is found on the ECG. This patient's complaints are most likely the result of

(A) prolonged symptoms of menopause
(B) masked depression
(C) a paraneoplastic syndrome
(D) apathetic hyperthyroidism
(E) ectopic cortisol production

10. Hyperparathyroidism in the elderly most commonly presents as

(A) asymptomatic hypercalcemia
(B) bone pain
(C) renal calculi
(D) peptic ulcer disease
(E) depression

11. The diagnosis of primary osteoporosis relies on the exclusion of all other possible underlying causes of osteoporosis. Inherited or acquired abnormalities that must be excluded in the diagnosis include all of the following EXCEPT

(A) chronic treatment with corticosteroids
(B) Paget's disease
(C) multiple myeloma
(D) hypogonadism
(E) idiopathic hypercalciuria

12. Hyperosmolar nonketotic coma is a life-threatening event that primarily occurs in elderly patients. The most important measure in the acute treatment of hyperosmolar nonketotic coma is

(A) intravenous hydration
(B) intravenous insulin
(C) intravenous sodium bicarbonate
(D) intravenous vasopressors
(E) subcutaneous heparin

13. All of the following statements about treatment of Paget's disease are true EXCEPT

(A) asymptomatic disease does not require treatment
(B) nonsteroidal anti-inflammatory drugs alone are appropriate therapy for Paget's disease involving the hip
(C) the serum alkaline phosphatase level reflects disease activity and response to treatment
(D) ectopic bone growth around a prosthesis precludes total joint replacement
(E) chronic calcitonin treatment causes decreased bone resorption and formation

14. A 78-year-old hypertensive diabetic patient uses 30 units of NPH insulin and 15 units of regular insulin each morning. Laboratory testing over the last year has revealed slowly increasing proteinuria and worsening renal function (a recent serum creatinine level is 2.8 mg/dl). Which of the following actions is most appropriate for the management of this patient?

(A) Switch from single (A.M. only) to split (A.M. and P.M.) dosing of insulin
(B) Discontinue the use of NPH insulin
(C) Avoid or discontinue the use of diuretics
(D) Decrease the total insulin dosage
(E) Instruct the patient to check the urine daily for evidence of ketones

15. An 80-year-old hypertensive man is found to have a serum potassium level of 5.8 mg/dl on routine electrolyte screening. This finding could be the result of all of the following underlying factors EXCEPT

(A) normal aging
(B) diabetes mellitus with mild renal impairment
(C) diuretic therapy
(D) multiple myeloma
(E) renovascular hypertension

16. An 80-year-old man complains of painful enlargement of his left breast. All of the following conditions could be the cause of gynecomastia in this patient EXCEPT

(A) cirrhosis
(B) digoxin treatment
(C) pituitary neoplasm
(D) pulmonary neoplasm
(E) hypothyroidism

17. A 70-year-old man complains of the recent onset of impotence, decreased libido, and breast tenderness and enlargement. He also has expressed some milky fluid from his right breast. What is the most likely cause of his complaints?

(A) Diabetes mellitus
(B) Depression
(C) Pituitary tumor
(D) Digoxin treatment
(E) Male breast carcinoma

Directions: The groups of questions below consist of an introductory premise or case data followed by four statements that pertain to the information given. Indicate whether each statement is **true** or **false**.

Questions 18–21

Thyroid function tests are performed in a seriously ill 80-year-old man. The following laboratory results indicate that he likely has active thyroid disease.

18. Elevated serum T_4, elevated serum T_3, and normal serum TSH

19. Decreased serum T_4, decreased serum T_3, and normal serum TSH

20. Decreased serum T_4, decreased serum T_3, and increased serum TSH

21. Elevated serum T_4, decreased serum T_3, and normal serum TSH

Questions 22–25

The following are reasons that chlorpropamide is not a preferred oral hypoglycemic agent for treating elderly diabetic patients.

22. It frequently produces hypoglycemia in older diabetic patients

23. It decreases the renal GFR

24. It produces severe hyponatremia in some elderly diabetic patients

25. It is less effective treatment of these patients than other sulfonylurea drugs

Questions 26–29

Lung cancer primarily is a disease of elderly smokers. Although most lung cancer patients are seen first because of pulmonary symptoms, others come to the physician's attention because of symptoms secondary to ectopic substance secretion by the neoplasm (paraneoplastic syndromes). Such symptom complexes include the following.

26. Complaints of nervousness, weight loss, weakness, and decreased libido combined with findings of tachycardia, gynecomastia, and tremor

27. Complaints of muscle weakness, easy bruising, hyperpigmentation, and excessive thirst combined with findings of hypertension and glucose intolerance

28. Complaints of lethargy, confusion, headache, and vomiting combined with findings of hyponatremia and low BUN

29. Complaints of constipation and frequent urination combined with findings of hypercalcemia and hypophosphatemia

Questions 30–33

A 70-year-old woman is found, on several biochemical screenings, to have a serum calcium level ranging between 11 mg/dl and 12 mg/dl. The only symptoms that can be attributed to this patient's hypercalcemia are weakness and an increased feeling of fatigue. After history, physical examination, and specific screening procedures do not disclose a possible nonparathyroid source of the hypercalcemia, it is assumed that this patient has an adenoma or hyperplasia of the parathyroid glands. The following therapeutic options can be offered to this patient.

30. Oral estrogen–progestin therapy
31. Oral phosphate therapy
32. Thiazide diuretic therapy
33. Surgical removal of parathyroid tissue

Case 1: Questions 34–45

Questions 34–37

A 75-year-old woman is seen because of a 10-month history of gradually deteriorating memory and hearing, weight gain, and increasing dyspnea and chest pain. Initial examination of this patient reveals a weak pulse of 52 beats/min, a puffy pale face with thickened doughy skin, a coarse voice, and a delayed relaxation phase of the deep tendon reflexes. Laboratory blood evaluation would be expected to show elevation of the following values.

34. Serum CK and LDH levels
35. Serum TSH level
36. Fasting blood sugar level
37. Serum cholesterol level

Questions 38–41

The findings on physical examination and laboratory evaluation of this patient lead to the decision to initiate thyroid replacement therapy. The following issues should be addressed in the treatment of this patient.

38. It may be best to hospitalize this patient for initiation of the therapy
39. Adrenal function should be assessed at the time that replacement begins
40. The appropriate initial daily dosage should not exceed 0.025 mg/day
41. The best thyroid replacement preparation is desiccated thyroid extract

Questions 42–45

Evidence of atherosclerotic heart disease in this patient raises the following issues concerning angina in the setting of hypothyroidism that requires replacement therapy.

42. A paradoxical improvement in angina can occur with thyroid replacement
43. Nitrate therapy is safe and well tolerated in these patients
44. A reversible cardiomyopathy is believed to occur in some hypothyroid patients
45. Thyroid hormone effects on the myocardium are mediated through the adrenergic receptors

Questions 46–49

The following patients are good candidates for postmenopausal estrogen replacement therapy cycled with progesterone.

46. A 78-year-old thin, healthy black woman with symptoms of atrophic vaginitis
47. A 76-year-old obese, hypertensive black woman with supraclavicular soft tissue fullness, radiographic evidence of vertebral osteopenia, and new glucose intolerance
48. A 70-year-old white woman with hot flashes and chronic symptoms of depression
49. A 65-year-old thin, small white woman who had a hysterectomy 20 years ago for uterine cancer and who had been taking oral estrogen but stopped recently because she is afraid of side effects

ANSWERS AND EXPLANATIONS

1. The answer is C. Routine serum calcium measurement has led to the increased discovery of primary hyperparathyroidism in older adults. Often there are no symptoms, just hypercalcemia. When symptoms are present, they are highly varied and generally related to the effects of hypercalcemia or to the effects of increased PTH on bones and joints. Symptoms and signs due to hypercalcemia include CNS effects (e.g., memory loss, depression, lethargy), neuromuscular effects (e.g., proximal muscle weakness), cardiovascular effects (e.g., hypertension), renal effects (e.g., polyuria, nephrocalcinosis), and gastrointestinal effects (e.g., constipation). Symptoms and signs related to increased PTH are less common and include bone pain and bone cysts due to osteitis fibrosa cystica.

2. The answer is A. Diabetic neuropathy is common in elderly patients who have a long history of diabetes and severe hyperglycemia. Autonomic neuropathy occurs less commonly than peripheral polyneuropathy (i.e., distal, bilateral sensory changes), but it can cause severe disability in some patients. The most frequent complications involve the cardiovascular, gastrointestinal, and genitourinary systems. Postural hypotension and tachycardia are common cardiovascular findings in patients with diabetic autonomic neuropathy. Delayed gastric emptying (gastroparesis) and episodic nocturnal diarrhea are common gastrointestinal complications. Genitourinary involvement is particularly problematic and is characterized by bladder dysfunction and urinary retention as well as impotence and retrograde ejaculation in men. Hypoglycemic reactions may become severe because the early adrenergic warning signals (i.e., sweating, tremor, palpitations) may not be perceived by a diabetic patient with autonomic neuropathy.

3. The answer is D. Hyponatremia in elderly patients frequently can be traced to an ectopic source of ADH—usually bronchogenic carcinoma. Other tumors (e.g., pancreatic, prostatic, and bladder carcinomas) as well as certain CNS disorders (e.g., infection) and pulmonary disorders (e.g., tuberculosis, pneumonia) also can cause inappropriate secretion of ADH and, thus, hyponatremia. Diabetes insipidus is characterized by the opposite effect (i.e., hypernatremia) due to ADH insufficiency (central diabetes insipidus) or to renal unresponsiveness to ADH (nephrogenic diabetes insipidus). Impaired thirst also can lead to hypernatremia; this rare occurrence is restricted to cases of coma or severe stroke, which render patients incapable of communicating thirst. Diabetic ketoacidosis and mannitol administration can cause an osmotic diuresis—another mechanism for producing hypernatremia.

4. The answer is C. The diagnosis of hypothyroidism is made readily by the finding of a reduced free T_4 index. To confirm that the hypothyroidism is due to thyroid disease, however, requires the additional finding of an increased serum TSH level. Hypothyroidism that is caused by an organic defect in the pituitary gland or hypothalamus is associated with a decreased free T_4 index and a normal or decreased serum TSH level. Serum T_3 levels often are in the normal range in hypothyroid patients and, even if reduced somewhat, do not aid in the diagnosis of primary hypothyroidism. When thyroid antibody levels are associated with hypothyroid disease, they are increased, not decreased. An elevated free T_4 index is diagnostic of hyperthyroidism, not hypothyroidism.

In the elderly, hypothyroidism may cause excessive sleepiness, memory loss, hearing impairment, and psychomotor retardation. Elderly hypothyroid patients who present with these symptoms often are believed to be suffering from senile dementia when, in fact, their disorder is entirely reversible.

5. The answer is C. Numerous factors can lead to erectile dysfunction, especially in elderly men. Depression as well as a variety of drugs (e.g., antihypertensives, antipsychotics, alcohol) and chronic illnesses (e.g., cardiovascular disease, diabetes) are important causative factors in this age-group. Endocrine disorders also must be considered, however. The primary endocrine causes of impotence include pituitary disorders or testicular disorders that cause testosterone insufficiency as well as hyperprotactinemia, estrogen excess (e.g., due to liver disease), and hyperthyroidism. When evaluating hypogonadism as the cause of impotence, it is necessary to determine whether the disorder lies in the hypothalamus, the pituitary gland, or the testis. A decreased testosterone level with a normal or increased LH level indicates that hypogonadism is due to a primary testicular disorder. A decreased testosterone level with a low LH level implies that there is a disorder of the hypothalamus or pituitary gland.

6. The answer is D. Serum calcium levels may be elevated in elderly patients as a result of many diseases and conditions besides primary hyperparathyroidism. The differential diagnosis of nonparathyroid hypercalcemia in the elderly should include certain malignancies (especially bronchogenic carcinoma, breast carcinoma, and multiple myeloma), hyperthyroidism, and certain drugs. In bronchogenic carcinoma, the underlying cause of hypercalcemia is believed to be the secretion of a PTH-like substance by malignant tissues. This "ectopic hyperparathyroidism" is not noted in breast carcinoma; the cause of hypercalcemia with this malignancy is not certain. In multiple myeloma, there is increased osteoclast activity induced by myeloma cells. Bone resorption is increased in patients with hyperthyroidism, which is believed to be the cause of hypercalcemia noted in many hyperthyroid patients. Ingestion of large amounts of calcium-containing antacids also can lead to increased serum calcium levels; this potential cause should not be overlooked in elderly patients, who are likely to self-medicate with these drugs. Although thiazide diuretics can promote hypercalcemia in some patients, loop diuretics (furosemide, ethacrynic acid, bumetanide) increase calciuria and, thus, do not promote hypercalcemia.

7. The answer is D. This patient is a candidate for therapy with a sulfonylurea drug (e.g., acetohexamide, chlorpropamide, glyburide, tolbutamide). These oral hypoglycemic agents are used to treat type II diabetes in patients who cannot be treated by dietary control or insulin therapy. Sulfanilamide is one of the sulfonamides, which are antimicrobial agents. The sulfonylureas were developed after the discovery, in the 1940s, that some sulfonamide drugs had a hypoglycemic effect. Today's antimicrobial sulfonamides are not likely to cause hypoglycemia, but they may increase the hypoglycemic effects of the sulfonylureas.

8. The answer is B. Osteoporosis is a disease of bone loss, which is extremely common in elderly women. A host of factors contribute to the process of bone loss in older women. Bone loss begins at some point after maximal skeletal mass is attained in early adulthood. Clearly, with greater bone density at maturity, there is a smaller percentage loss of bone with aging. Epidemiologic studies have shown that women of short stature and northern European heritage tend to have the lightest skeletons and a high incidence of osteoporosis later in life. An important risk factor that can be prevented is estrogen deficiency following menopause. With estrogen replacement, postmenopausal women do not experience accelerated bone loss due to lack of estrogen. Sporadic factors that contribute to an increased rate of bone loss include cigarette smoking, heavy alcohol consumption, low dietary calcium, and sedentary lifestyle. Obesity is recognized as a protective factor, possibly due to increased loading stress to the skeleton and to increased conversion of adrenal androgens to estrogens in fat tissue.

9. The answer is D. Thyrotoxicosis is common among elderly hyperthyroid patients. Weight loss and heat intolerance are classic features of thyrotoxicosis in patients of all ages. However, listlessness, depression, and atrial fibrillation are characteristic of apathetic hyperthyroidism—a variant of hyperthyroidism that is seen predominantly in the elderly. Symptoms of congestive heart failure also are common in apathetic hyperthyroidism. In elderly hyperthyroid patients, it is not uncommon to find only elevated serum T_3 levels—so-called "T_3 toxicosis." Further, one-third or more of elderly patients with thyrotoxicosis have no palpable thyroid gland abnormality. Perimenopausal symptoms are unlikely in a 65-year-old woman. Although this patient's complaints and mood could suggest masked depression, the other symptoms and signs (e.g., heat intolerance, atrial fibrillation) are more indicative of apathetic hyperthyroidism. Heat intolerance is not a characteristic symptom of paraneoplastic syndromes or ectopic cortisol production.

10. The answer is A. Primary hyperparathyroidism is a relatively common problem in people who are over the age of 60. This disorder is most commonly discovered on routine serum chemistry screening, which reveals an elevated calcium level. Osteitis fibrosa cystica, renal calculi, peptic ulcers, and depression certainly are common features of symptomatic disease, which is associated with persistent serum calcium levels exceeding 11 mg/dl. Mood changes as well as arthralgias, myalgias, and generalized aching are common clinical manifestations in elderly patients with hyperparathyroidism, which may occur before the other, more obvious, features.

11. The answer is B. The differential diagnosis of primary osteoporosis (referred to as involutional osteoporosis when it occurs in association with aging) is based largely on exclusion of other disorders that can cause or contribute to bone loss. In most patients with a vertebral compression fracture, osteoporosis should be suspected and can be confirmed on the basis of the clinical data collected. It is important to consider the other potential causes or contributing factors at this time. Some of these can be eliminated fairly easily on the basis of the initial history, physical examination, and laboratory procedures. Chronic administration of pharmacologic doses of glucocorticoids is a common cause of secondary osteoporosis. Testosterone deficiency and estrogen deficiency (after menopause) are associated with an accelerated and intensified loss of bone. At least 5% of patients who present with vertebral compression fractures exhibit hypercalciuria. These patients usually do not have other features of secondary causes of hypercalciuria and, thus, are considered to have idiopathic hypercalciuria. Multiple myeloma usually can be eliminated from the differential diagnosis on the basis of a normal hematocrit and erythrocyte sedimentation rate and the absence of characteristic monoclonal proteins in the serum and urine. Paget's disease does not cause or contribute to generalized bone loss; this disease is characterized by focal areas where bone remodeling and bone resorption occur. Radiographic studies of typical lesions show bone that is rewoven by both processes.

12. The answer is A. Hyperosmolar nonketotic coma occurs mainly in elderly patients with type II diabetes—often before the disorder has been diagnosed. The hyperglycemia often develops over a period of days and leads to osmotic diuresis, which causes progressive dehydration and decline in mental status. Focal and reversible neurologic signs may be mistaken for stroke in an elderly patient. In the acute treatment of hyperosmolar nonketotic coma, the first and most important step is fluid replacement. The preferred initial treatment is intravenous administration of several liters of 1/2 N saline; if hypotension is present, isotonic saline should be infused instead. Vasopressor agents should not be given until the intravascular volume has been replenished. Rapid intravascular volume replacement may help to prevent thrombosis, and arterial and venous thromboses are relatively common complications. Low-dose insulin administration is an important step in the early treatment of hyperosmolar coma, but the insulin deficiency is not as profound as the intravascular fluid deficiency. Bicarbonate usually is not required.

13. The answer is D. Paget's disease is a disorder of bone remodeling that occurs commonly in people over the age of 40; the incidence may be greater than 10% in those who reach the age of 80. Paget's disease occurs commonly in the United States, Europe, and Australia but rarely in the Middle and Far East. Its cause is unknown, but it may be due to an osteoclastic viral infection that remains dormant for years before causing clinical manifestations. Active bone resorption induces new bone formation, and typical lesions show bone rewoven by both processes. Although most cases involve local disease that remains asymptomatic and requires no treatment, patients who have extensive disease with pain, nerve compression, bone deformities, pathologic fractures, or high-output congestive heart failure often benefit from specific treatment. Patients with degenerative joint disease resulting from Paget's involvement of periarticular bone also may benefit from such treatment, although they often improve simply with nonsteroidal anti-inflammatory treatment of the joint pain. Total joint replacement is an option for patients with severe joint damage from Paget's disease; ectopic bone formation may occur but often does not interfere with prosthesis function.

The available treatments (i.e., calcitonin, diphosphonates, mithramycin) act primarily by inhibiting osteoclast function and differentiation. Chronic calcitonin use decreases both bone resorption and formation. The serum alkaline phosphatase level falls in response to successful treatment and generally reflects the degree of disease activity.

14. The answer is D. About half of the amount of endogenous or exogenous insulin that is delivered to the liver is degraded in a single pass through the hepatic circulation. Insulin then is filtered through the kidney, where it is reabsorbed and further metabolized. Thus, the kidney is an important site of insulin metabolism. In fact, diminished renal function appears to have as great an effect as hepatic disease on insulin clearance from the plasma. Even a normal liver cannot compensate for the decreased catabolic function of the kidney. This patient's slowly increasing proteinuria and gradually declining renal function strongly suggest that she is in the early stages of diabetic nephropathy. It is appropriate to expect that this patient's diminished renal function has resulted in an increased plasma concentration of insulin due to decreased metabolism and clearance by the kidney. Therefore, the best action to be taken at this time is to decrease this patient's total insulin dosage. As a diabetic patient becomes progressively more uremic, peripheral resistance to insulin action also occurs, which can worsen glucose tolerance.

15. The answer is E. A person with renovascular hypertension would be expected to have elevated renin, angiotensin, and aldosterone levels due to the renal ischemia, which would result in sodium retention and hypokalemia, not hyperkalemia. In the elderly, there is a decreased response of the renin-angiotensin-aldosterone axis to typical stimuli such as sodium restriction and upright posture. Therefore, a mildly elevated serum potassium level may be a normal finding in an elderly patient. Hyporeninemic hypoaldosteronism also is more common in older patients; a typical setting would be a diabetic patient with renal functional impairment that is not severe enough to explain an elevation in the serum potassium level. Multiple myeloma with light chain nephropathy and interstitial nephritis are other renal causes of this syndrome. The use of potassium-sparing diuretics and the presence of primary adrenocortical insufficiency are other factors to be considered.

16. The answer is E. Gynecomastia can be found at autopsy in up to 40% of elderly men. Typically, it is asymptomatic and undiscovered unless rapid enlargement causes pain or tenderness. The most common cause of gynecomastia in any age-group is a disturbance of the balanced effects of estrogenic and androgenic hormones on breast tissue. However, a primary breast malignancy always must be considered, particularly if breast enlargement is unilateral.

Typical causes of gynecomastia include treatment with drugs such as spironolactone, digoxin, cimetidine, and CNS-acting agents. Systemic diseases such as cirrhosis, thyrotoxicosis (not hypothyroidism), and renal failure can alter estrogen metabolism and cause gynecomastia. More worrisome and relatively more common causes in the elderly are tumors that secrete estrogen (e.g., adrenal tumors), HCG (e.g., lung and hepatic carcinomas), or prolactin (e.g., pituitary tumors). Testicular neoplasms become progressively less common after adolescence.

The evaluation of an elderly patient with gynecomastia typically includes a complete history and physical examination, which focus on identifying underlying drug treatments or systemic illnesses that might explain the syndrome. Chest x-ray as well as androgen, estrogen, HCG, prolactin, and LH assays would be appropriate screening tests performed in the initial evaluation.

17. The answer is C. The only disorder listed that causes impotence, gynecomastia, and galactorrhea is a pituitary tumor. The typical situation is an elderly man who presents with impotence and decreased libido as manifestations of a prolactin-secreting tumor. Prolactin is associated with defective gonadotropin and testosterone secretion, which causes impotence. Gynecomastia and galactorrhea also may occur in some cases due to disturbance of the balanced effects of estrogen and androgen on breast tissue.

Measurement of serum prolactin is important in the evaluation of a patient with this syndrome; the finding of an elevated prolactin level should lead to brain CT or MRI scanning to look for a pituitary macroadenoma. Failure to identify a macroadenoma does not necessarily rule out a pituitary cause (e.g., a microadenoma too small to be visualized or idiopathic hypersecretion of prolactin). Nonpituitary causes of hyperprolactinemia also must be sought, such as various drugs, systemic diseases, and hypothalamic inflammatory or neoplastic disorders.

Pituitary causes of hyperprolactinemia often are treated medically, with bromocriptine (a dopamine agonist), rather than surgically. Bromocriptine suppresses pituitary secretion of prolactin and restores potency in most patients; in many cases, it also shrinks macroadenomas so that surgery can be avoided.

18–21. The answers are: 18-T, 19-F, 20-T, 21-F. Euthyroid sick syndrome is the name given to a variety of conditions characterized by abnormal results on thyroid function testing in the setting of severe illness that is not thyroid-related. Patients with euthyroid sick syndrome can appear to have either hyperthyroidism or hypothyroidism on laboratory testing due to increased or decreased TBG levels or impaired peripheral conversion of T_4 to T_3. TBG levels can be increased in certain chronic illnesses (e.g., cirrhosis) and can lead to increased serum T_4 levels, as can impaired conversion of T_4 to T_3.

In the first set of laboratory results, the elevated serum T_4 level in association with an elevated serum T_3 level suggests hyperthyroidism rather than the euthyroid sick syndrome. Most laboratories do not have tests for serum TSH level that are sensitive enough to distinguish between euthyroid and hyperthyroid status. The elevated serum T_3 level is the best proof of hyperthyroidism in this situation, since impaired T_4 conversion in the euthyroid sick state would lead to a low or normal T_3 level, and potential TBG abnormalities also would not elevate the serum T_3 level.

In the second set of laboratory results, the decreased serum T_4 level in association with a decreased serum T_3 level suggests the euthyroid sick syndrome rather than hypothyroidism because the serum TSH is normal. An increased serum TSH is the most sensitive test for hypothyroidism, even in this setting; the TSH level does not rise in response to a low serum T_3 level in the absence of hypothyroidism. Presumably, the serum T_4 level is low due to a decreased TBG level (a T_3 resin uptake or free T_4 index determination could be used to show this). The decreased serum T_3 level is most likely due to impaired peripheral conversion of T_4 to T_3. For unknown reasons, the mortality rate is extremely high for euthyroid sick patients with low serum T_4 levels.

The decreased serum T_4 and T_3 levels in association with an increased serum TSH level (third set of results) are most suggestive of hypothyroidism because of the increased serum TSH. In some cases, hypothyroid patients may have low T_4 levels with normal T_3 levels, since T_3 production and peripheral conversion of T_4 to T_3 are enhanced in hypothyroidism.

In the fourth set of laboratory results, the elevated serum T_4 level suggests hyperthyroidism, but the low serum T_3 level indicates that either an increased TBG level or impaired conversion of T_4 to T_3 is the reason for the high T_4 level; both of these abnormalities can be found in euthyroid sick syndrome. To make a diagnosis of hyperthyroidism in this situation, it would be necessary to show either an elevated serum T_3 or an elevated free T_4 index (reflecting a true increase in serum T_4 as well as in TBG) accompanied by a normal, not low, T_3 level.

22–25. The answers are: 22-T, 23-F, 24-T, 25-F. Sulfonylurea drugs account for almost all cases of drug-induced hypoglycemia in diabetic patients over 60 years of age. Chlorpropamide—the oldest sulfonylurea drug available, with the longest duration of action (30–36 hours)—accounts for nearly 50% of all sulfonylurea-related hypoglycemia episodes, which can be life threatening in elderly patients. Approximately 4% of diabetic patients taking chlorpropamide develop a syndrome of inappropriate ADH secretion, which manifests as severe hyponatremia. Elderly patients, patients with congestive heart failure, and patients who are taking diuretics are particularly predisposed to the hyponatremic effect of chlorpropamide. All of the sulfonylurea drugs generally are considered to be equal in efficacy. Chlorpropamide, like all sulfonylurea drugs, is contraindicated in patients with renal insufficiency, due to the important role of the kidneys in the excretion of this drug and its metabolites; however, sulfonylureas are not known to cause a decrease in the renal GFR.

26–29. The answers are: 26-F, 27-T, 28-T, 29-T. Some lung cancer patients come to the physician's attention because of symptoms relating to ectopic substance production by the neoplasm. Such paraneoplastic syndromes have been described in association with ectopic secretion of ACTH, ADH, and a PTH-like substance.

Ectopic ACTH secretion leads to clinical manifestations of glucocorticoid and mineralocorticoid excess. Patients present with features of Cushing's syndrome, including muscle wasting and weakness, effects of sodium retention (hypertension, peripheral edema), and decreased glucose tolerance, which results in symptoms of diabetes mellitus (polyuria, polydipsia, weight loss). Hyperpigmentation of the skin also occurs due to increased MSH activity that accompanies the increased secretion of ACTH.

Ectopic ADH secretion leads to clinical manifestations relating to hyponatremia. Patients present with lethargy, confusion, headache, decreased appetite, nausea, and vomiting. With severe degrees of hyponatremia, convulsions may occur.

Some solid tumors can secrete a humoral substance that has most of the bone and renal actions of PTH, even though actual PTH levels are suppressed. Ectopic PTH-like substance secretion leads to clinical manifestations of hypercalcemia. Patients present with constipation, frequent urination, and arthralgia. The high serum calcium level often is accompanied by a low serum phosphate level in these patients, similar to the clinical picture of primary hyperparathyroidism. Renal bicarbonate loss is not seen, however.

Excessive secretion of thyroid hormone leads to a variety of clinical manifestations of hypermetabolism. Patients present with such features as nervousness, tremor, weakness and muscle wasting, weight loss (despite increased appetite), decreased libido, gynecomastia, cardiac arrhythmias, and palpitations. Pulmonary neoplasms are not known to produce thyroid hormone.

30–33. The answers are: 30-T, 31-T, 32-F, 33-T. Several drug treatment options exist for a patient with a long history of only mild to moderate hypercalcemia with minimal symptoms. Finding a drug that is effective may take some trial and error, however. The patient should be aware, ahead of time, that long-term drug therapy for hypercalcemia can produce serious side effects and may not be the best choice if there is good reason to suspect a parathyroid source (e.g., adenoma, hyperplasia), which can be eradicated with surgery.

Mild to moderate hypercalcemia in a postmenopausal woman with primary hyperparathyroidism often can be managed successfully with oral estrogen–progestin combinations. Estrogen protects against bone resorption, which is an added benefit in this osteoporosis-prone population.

If hypercalcemia is not controlled with estrogen, oral phosphate (usually at an initial dose of 1–2 g/day) should be tried. Phosphate binds calcium, preventing its absorption. It is important to monitor serum calcium, phosphorus, and creatinine levels during treatment to gauge the effectiveness of the therapy and to guard against extraskeletal (e.g., renal) calcification.

A hypercalcemic patient who is not improved with phosphate may wish to consider surgery, if a diagnosis of primary hyperparathyroidism is confirmed. In a patient such as this with mild symptoms and hypercalcemia, surgical exploration usually uncovers a single adenoma, the excision of which is curative in almost all cases. If found, parathyroid hyperplasia can be treated by surgical excision of 3½ glands. The increased risk of surgery in the geriatric age-group must be considered when recommending such treatment.

Acute severe hypercalcemia (a serum calcium level exceeding 13 mg/dl) should be managed with hydration and forced diuresis with a loop diuretic (e.g., furosemide). Thiazide diuretics promote hypercalcemia and, thus, have no use in the treatment of this disorder, regardless of its severity.

34–37. The answers are: 34-T, 35-T, 36-F, 37-T. This patient presents with several of the classic signs and symptoms of hypothyroidism (weight gain, edema, husky voice) as well as features that are seen more commonly in elderly hypothyroid patients (diminished memory and hearing). Characteristic cardiovascular manifestations of hypothyroidism also are present in this patient (dyspnea, fatigue, angina, bradycardia, weak pulse).

Hematologic evaluation of a patient with such a broad range of hypothyroid manifestations is very likely to show an increased serum TSH level—the most reliable indication of primary hypothyroidism. (In the overwhelming majority of cases, hypothyroidism is caused by a lesion or malfunction of the thyroid gland.) Other biochemical abnormalities that are common in patients with moderate to severe hypothyroidism include an elevated serum cholesterol level as well as increased CK, LDH, and SGOT levels, which often are secondary to a myopathy and can lead to a misdiagnosis of myocardial infarction. The fasting blood sugar level often is decreased in hypothyroidism.

38–41. The answers are: 38-T, 39-F, 40-T, 41-F. Although hospitalization is not an absolute requirement, it is wise to hospitalize elderly patients for initiation of thyroid replacement therapy, particularly if there is a history of cardiovascular symptoms. Replacement with too high a dosage of thyroid hormone may precipitate angina, myocardial infarction, arrhythmia, or heart failure. The usual therapeutic amount (0.1–0.2 mg/day) would be unsuitable in this situation; usually, a dosage of 0.025 mg/day or less is preferred, although the amount must be individualized to each patient.

Meticulous attention also must be given to the rate of increase in thyroid replacement in these patients. Often, the maintenance dosage is 20%–40% smaller than that used in younger, healthier patients.

It is necessary to differentiate between primary and secondary hypothyroidism prior to the initiation of treatment, as an adrenal crisis may be precipitated by thyroid hormone replacement in the presence of adrenal failure from a pituitary adenoma. Although dessicated thyroid extract (a T_3-containing preparation) once was the standard of therapy, it has been replaced by levothyroxine (a T_4-containing preparation) as the therapy of choice. Preparations that contain T_3 are contraindicated because of their rapid absorption with rapidly peaking plasma concentrations, which can precipitate cardiac complications in older patients.

42–45. The answers are: 42-T, 43-F, 44-T, 45-F. The treatment of angina in an elderly hypothyroid patient requires great care. Studies of hypothyroid patients suggest that some of these patients develop a reversible cardiomyopathy involving asymmetric septal hypertrophy. Resolution of this abnormality would explain why some hypothyroid patients experience improvement (rather than worsening) of their angina on treatment with thyroid replacement alone. The use of nitrates to treat angina must be approached with great caution, as profound hypotension and syncope may develop. This particularly is a risk when blood and plasma volume are reduced, as can occur in myxedema. Because thyroxine's effect on the myocardium is independent of the adrenergic system, propranolol may not be effective for the prevention of angina in hypothyroid patients on replacement therapy.

46–49. The answers are: 46-T, 47-F, 48-F, 49-T. Despite the advantages of estrogen replacement therapy during the postmenopausal years, estrogen therapy remains controversial. Administration of estrogen is associated with an increased risk for thromboembolic disease; in addition, there is a demonstrated increase in the incidence of uterine malignancy in patients who are given estrogen not cycled with progesterone. Furthermore, conflicting data exist as to whether estrogen replacement increases or decreases the risk for development of breast cancer or atherosclerotic coronary artery disease. However, estrogen appears to be effective therapy for hot flashes (i.e., a vasomotor episode with sweating) and for atrophic vaginitis as well as effective prophylaxis against primary osteoporosis if given in the first 5 years after menopause. (Estrogens decrease the rate of calcium loss that is characteristic of menopause.)

A healthy black woman with atrophic vaginitis would likely benefit from estrogen replacement in the absence of any significant contraindications. Cycling with progesterone would decrease the risk of endometrial carcinoma, and a yearly Pap smear and pelvic, breast, and mammographic examination would be appropriate to monitor a patient on such treatment. Vaginal estrogen creams also are used in the treatment of atrophic vaginitis, but significant systemic absorption occurs with these preparations.

The hypertensive patient described here exhibits manifestations that could be attributed to Cushing's syndrome, and this etiology should be investigated before osteoporosis treatment is initiated. Obese black women ordinarily are at relatively low risk for significant osteopenia; secondary causes always should be considered, especially when the clinical setting is atypical.

Hot flashes associated with menopause typically are most troubling in the first 5 years after menopause. A 70-year-old woman who complains of hot flashes, therefore, may not be experiencing the effects of estrogen deficiency. The associated depression would not be expected to respond to estrogen replacement, so there is no good reason to administer estrogen to this patient.

An elderly woman who had a hysterectomy much earlier in her life is a good candidate for cycled hormone therapy. The accelerated bone loss that occurs after menopause begins again when estrogen replacement is stopped. In addition, the elderly woman described here is white, lean, and small—all factors that further increase her risk for osteoporosis. She has not suffered evident complications during her long treatment with estrogen. Therefore, this woman would benefit greatly from restarting estrogen therapy for protection against accelerated osteopenia. Her prior hysterectomy has eliminated the risk for uterine cancer as a complication of this treatment. Since her earlier treatment with estrogen was not complicated by side effects, it is appropriate to continue treatment with proper monitoring (as described above). The potential risks and benefits of estrogen replacement should be discussed with her.

10
Psychiatric Disorders

QUESTIONS

Directions: Each question below contains five suggested answers. Choose the **one best** response to each question.

1. The early phase (1–3 years) of Alzheimer's disease may be characterized by all of the following signs and symptoms EXCEPT

(A) anomia
(B) short-term memory impairment
(C) difficulty in abstraction
(D) impaired judgment
(E) incontinence

2. Alcohol abuse is misdiagnosed and underdiagnosed in the elderly. Certain findings in an elderly patient should alert the physician to a possible alcohol abuse problem. All of the following conditions are associated with alcohol abuse in the elderly EXCEPT

(A) depression
(B) incontinence
(C) hostility
(D) diarrhea
(E) hypothermia

3. The most appropriate antidepressant for an 85-year-old woman who suffers from a postural blood pressure drop is

(A) amitriptyline
(B) imipramine
(C) nortriptyline
(D) doxepin
(E) maprotiline

4. Each of the following conditions commonly seen in elderly patients is a well-established side effect of one or more of the phenothiazines EXCEPT

(A) osteopenia
(B) leukopenia
(C) gynecomastia
(D) agitation
(E) orthostatic hypotension

5. All of the following statements concerning elderly opiate addicts are true EXCEPT

(A) they generally are addicted to other nonopiate drugs
(B) they have a history of heavy smoking
(C) they have a reasonable degree of control over their use of opiates
(D) they generally are active participants in a methadone maintenance program
(E) they have a strong genetic advantage toward long life

6. Depression in the elderly may be caused by all of the following drugs EXCEPT

(A) reserpine
(B) levodopa
(C) propranolol
(D) prednisone
(E) digoxin

7. Routine prelithium treatment evaluation in the elderly should include all of the following items EXCEPT

(A) serum creatinine level
(B) baseline TSH level
(C) baseline ECG
(D) CBC
(E) liver function testing

8. Immediately following the death of a spouse, a person is most likely to

(A) experience a sense of profound loss and despair
(B) experience a sense of emotional numbness and denial
(C) take on attributes of the spouse in an effort at reclamation
(D) experience a sense of yearning and longing
(E) experience a sense of deep affection for the deceased person

9. The leading cause of significant cognitive impairment among the elderly is

(A) advancing age
(B) declining intelligence
(C) dementia
(D) vitamin deficiency
(E) depression

10. The most common irreversible dementia of later life is a manifestation of

(A) Alzheimer's disease
(B) Creutzfeldt-Jakob disease
(C) Parkinson's disease
(D) head trauma
(E) alcoholism

11. A 72-year-old woman enters the hospital. She has lost 15 pounds and says she has no interest in eating. The physical examination and laboratory findings are normal. She has been awakening at 5 A.M. for several months and cannot fall back to sleep. She says she has been feeling anxious and helpless since her husband died 3 years ago. A reasonable medication to prescribe for her would be

(A) an antipsychotic
(B) a tricyclic antidepressant
(C) a minor tranquilizer
(D) lithium
(E) a β blocker

12. Which of the following factors is most contributory to late-onset alcoholism?

(A) Family history of alcoholism
(B) Psychosocial stress
(C) Associated illicit drug abuse
(D) Personality disorder
(E) History of previous alcohol-related problems

13. All patients who present with significant cognitive impairment should undergo a comprehensive evaluation that includes all of the following tests EXCEPT

(A) lumbar puncture
(B) serology (VDRL)
(C) thyroid function testing
(D) vitamin B_{12} and folate levels
(E) erythrocyte sedimentation rate

14. Prophylaxis for recurrent mania in the older patient usually is best managed with

(A) lithium carbonate alone
(B) an antipsychotic drug in combination with lithium carbonate
(C) an antipsychotic drug alone
(D) a benzodiazepine
(E) carbamazepine

15. Major hypotheses regarding the etiology and pathogenesis of Alzheimer's disease include all of the following EXCEPT

(A) changes in protein metabolism
(B) neurochemical aberrations
(C) cerebrovascular vasoconstriction
(D) prion (subviral particle) infection
(E) accumulation of metals

Questions 16–18

A 65-year-old business executive with advanced cirrhosis of the liver and a history of alcohol abuse claims that he does not have a problem with drinking and can quit at any time.

16. The primary defense mechanism that he is using is

(A) projection
(B) denial
(C) rationalization
(D) reaction formation
(E) isolation of affect

17. At other times he says that he drinks only because of the constant nagging of his wife. This defense mechanism is best identified as

(A) rationalization
(B) regression
(C) sublimation
(D) reaction formation
(E) isolation of affect

18. Eventually this patient quits drinking but continues to suffer from advanced cirrhosis of the liver. In spite of his obvious abdominal distension from ascites he tells everyone how happy he is to have cirrhosis since it has led to the cessation of his drinking. The defense mechanism he is using is best identified as

(A) projection
(B) denial
(C) counterphobic behavior
(D) reaction formation
(E) isolation of affect

Questions 19–21

A 59-year-old woman with a history of chronic paranoid schizophrenia has become acutely agitated, and treatment with 40 mg of trifluoperazine is started. After 3 weeks, the woman is observed sitting motionless and unresponsive in a chair all day. When helped to walk, she has a shuffling gait.

19. What is the most likely diagnosis?

(A) Exacerbation of the schizophrenic disorder with a catatonic stupor
(B) Hypothyroidism secondary to the trifluoperazine
(C) Akinesia secondary to the trifluoperazine
(D) Major depressive disorder with psychomotor retardation
(E) Apathy and dependency secondary to chronic hospitalization

20. What is the most appropriate initial step in treating this woman?

(A) Increasing the dosage of trifluoperazine
(B) Encouraging the patient to participate in ward activities
(C) Adding an antiparkinsonian drug
(D) Decreasing the dosage of trifluoperazine and adding a thyroid hormone
(E) Adding a tricyclic antidepressant

21. If the first treatment approach is unsuccessful, what is the next step?

(A) Changing to a different antipsychotic
(B) Changing to a different antidepressant
(C) Adding a stimulant such as dextroamphetamine
(D) Increasing the thyroid hormone
(E) Administering ECT

Questions 22–24

A 70-year old male alcoholic who is enrolled in an outpatient program presents with insomnia and decreased appetite. He continues to have periodic heavy drinking bouts followed by prolonged periods of abstinence. His major complaints are depression and alienation from family members because of his alcohol problem.

22. Which of the following medications would best relieve this patient's symptoms?

(A) Disulfiram
(B) Diazepam
(C) Chlorpromazine
(D) Flurazepam
(E) Doxepin

23. What is the next most appropriate step in this patient's treatment?

(A) Group therapy and socialization
(B) Referral to an inpatient alcohol rehabilitation program
(C) Psychiatric workup and psychological evaluation
(D) Hospitalization
(E) Follow-up nursing home visits

24. The patient presents with tachycardia, fever (102.5° F), urinary retention, and hot, dry skin. He is presently on 50 mg of doxepin daily. After inserting a Foley catheter and obtaining appropriate cultures, the physician should

(A) administer 25 mg of bethanechol
(B) begin parenteral administration of thiamine
(C) obtain a urine drug screen
(D) check for use of over-the-counter cold and allergy medications
(E) decrease the dosage of doxepin to 25 mg daily

Directions: The groups of questions below consist of an introductory premise or case data followed by four statements that pertain to the information given. Indicate whether each statement is **true** or **false**.

Questions 25–28

Toxic effects of over-the-counter drugs rarely are recognized until organ damage occurs. Over-the-counter drug use by the elderly can be described accurately by the following statements.

25. Elderly over-the-counter drug users consume significantly greater quantities of the remedies than younger people

26. Because of their lower cost and accessibility, over-the-counter drugs are used by the elderly instead of alcohol or prescribed drugs

27. Psychotherapeutic or substance abuse–oriented treatment programs are appropriate for over-the-counter drug users

28. Because of increased drug sensitivity with age, elderly patients are more prone to over-the-counter drug toxicity and dependence than younger people

Questions 29–32

The relationship between the noradrenergic system and Alzheimer's disease is characterized by the following statements.

29. Decreased cortical norepinephrine is a consistent finding in Alzheimer's disease

30. Aberrations in the cortical noradrenergic system in Alzheimer's disease probably are secondary phenomena related to severe cholinergic disease (acetylcholine deficiency)

31. Noradrenergic changes observed in patients with Alzheimer's disease correlate strongly with the clinical severity of the disease

32. Change in the noradrenergic system is a more sensitive indicator of the presence of Alzheimer's disease than is change in choline acetyltransferase

Questions 33–36

The following statements accurately describe the demographics of suicide among the elderly.

33. Suicide rates among elderly blacks and native Americans greatly exceed the national rate

34. Suicide occurs at a higher rate among the elderly than among young persons (between 13 and 22 years old)

35. Elderly people are likely to express suicidal ideation openly

36. The greatest number of successful suicides among women occur after the age of 55

Questions 37–40

Creutzfeldt-Jakob disease is a rare, fatal disorder of the CNS. The following statements describe hallmarks of Creutzfeldt-Jakob disease.

37. The disease is transmissible to nonhuman primates

38. Myoclonus occurs in most patients at some time in the disease

39. Clinical variations in Creutzfeldt-Jakob disease make it difficult to distinguish from Alzheimer's disease

40. The disease can result from growth hormone therapy

Questions 41–44

The elderly constitute a special population when addiction treatment strategies are considered. The following statements accurately describe treatment of the elderly alcoholic.

41. Because of their denial of an alcohol problem, older alcoholics are less responsive and more hostile to treatment than younger alcoholics

42. Senior citizen day programs and outpatient geriatric programs are appropriate facilities to treat the elderly alcoholic

43. Antidepressant medication may be effective in eliminating alcohol abuse in some elderly patients

44. Disulfiram is appropriately prescribed for older alcoholics

Questions 45–48

The following symptoms sometimes are treated with low-potency antipsychotic medications but, in fact, may be caused by these drugs.

45. Hallucinations

46. Confusion

47. Agitation

48. Emotional lability

Questions 49–52

Many of the over-the-counter drugs used by the elderly cause physical and psychological ailments. All of the following statements accurately describe the effects of over-the-counter drug abuse and dependence.

49. Laxative abuse can lead to hypokalemia and vitamin deficiencies

50. Of the analgesics, only aspirin has been linked with renal disease

51. Phenylpropanolamine can cause adverse reactions in patients taking MAO inhibitors

52. Calcium and magnesium found in antacids can produce psychiatric symptoms in the elderly

Questions 53–56

As a person with bipolar disorder ages, the following changes in the nature of the illness may occur.

53. Manic and depressive characteristics can overlap in the elderly

54. Both manic and depressive episodes diminish, and the disorder eventually "burns out"

55. The length of time between manic episodes lessens

56. The disorder often evolves into unipolar depression

Questions 57–60

The following antianxiety medications are appropriate for treating a 78-year-old elderly man with cirrhosis.

57. Diazepam

58. Lorazepam

59. Flurazepam

60. Oxazepam

Questions 61–64

Paraphrenia is a paranoid disorder in which the disturbance is not severe enough to justify a *DSM III-R* diagnosis. Characteristics of paraphrenia are summarized by the following statements.

61. Paraphrenia rarely is seen in older persons apart from other psychopathology

62. Patients with paraphrenia often respond to confrontation and clarification on the part of the therapist

63. Paraphrenia is appropriately treated with antipsychotic medication

64. Paraphrenia involves delusions that usually are persecutory and poorly systematized

ANSWERS AND EXPLANATIONS

1. The answer is E. Many features of early Alzheimer's disease suggest the diagnosis. Usually, there is impairment of short-term memory and then impairment of judgment. Personality, however, often is well preserved early in Alzheimer's disease. Among the other important early symptoms are anomia, or difficulty in naming objects, which is significant diagnostically in the absence of prior stroke, and difficulty in abstraction. Assessment of these clinical features requires asking the patient to name an object, to describe the meaning of a proverb, and to remember objects for several minutes. Incontinence, motor disorders, and gait disturbances early in the illness should prompt a search for normal pressure hydrocephalus as a cause of the memory loss.

2. The answer is C. Data regarding alcohol abuse in the elderly are inconsistent and unreliable. Physicians miss the diagnosis of alcoholism in 20% of older hospitalized patients because they present with complaints generally not indicative of substance abuse. Many conditions should alert the physician to possible alcohol abuse, including diarrhea, myopathy, incontinence, hypothermia, injuries, self-neglect, falls, and unusual behavior. Typically, older alcoholic patients tend to be less hostile than younger problem drinkers, as evidenced by lower scores on the psychopathic deviation, paranoia, and hypomania scales of the Minnesota Multiphasic Personality Inventory (MMPI). These patterns suggest reduced levels of hostility, distrust, and impulsiveness. Depression is a common feature of alcoholism in any age-group.

3. The answer is C. Orthostatic hypotension is a particularly significant side effect of antidepressants in older people because of the frequency and severity of falls that are caused by this effect of these drugs. Nortriptyline is the agent least likely to cause postural blood pressure drop. Orthostatic hypotension is a common side effect not only of tricyclic antidepressants but also of MAO inhibitors. Although nortriptyline is less likely to have an effect on blood pressure than the other drugs listed, it has significant anticholinergic effects, including dizziness, constipation, edema, and urinary retention, which often limit its use in older persons.

4. The answer is A. Phenothiazines are relatively safe drugs. They may, however, produce a number of side effects that are problematic in elderly persons. The best known of these side effects is tardive dyskinesia, a potentially irreversible condition involving involuntary movements of the oral–lingual–buccal musculature, the extremities, or both. In addition, phenothiazines can cause leukopenia, through a mechanism that is not understood fully, and gynecomastia and galactorrhea, due to the prolactin-stimulating effect of the drugs. A subjective sense of uneasiness and restlessness (akathisia) may occur and often is mistaken for psychotic agitation in a patient taking a phenothiazine. Akathisia may be inappropriately treated by increasing the dosage of the antipsychotic medication. Some phenothiazines (e.g., chlorpromazine, thioridazine) also may produce orthostatic hypotension because of their α-adrenergic blocking activity. This side effect can be particularly hazardous in elderly individuals who are prone to falling. Loss of bone or calcium is not a side effect of phenothiazine.

5. The answer is A. Most elderly opiate users are not addicted to nonopiate drugs, including alcohol. Alcohol-related health problems among addicts are rare for those over the age of 65. These persons generally have a history of tobacco use and have been heavy smokers during their lives; the use of tobacco probably will be the major cause of death for most of them. These addicts reach old age because they have some control over their drug abuse. Although they use drugs consistently, without long periods of abstinence, they are capable of using smaller amounts and saving the drug until later in the day. Many elderly opiate addicts participate in methadone programs, which not only contribute to their physical health and longevity, but also play a major role in their social lives. Longevity often is found in the family history of elderly opiate addicts.

6. The answer is E. Older people often take a host of medications; therefore, consideration must be given to the psychiatric side effects of the drugs that they take. The list of drugs producing psychiatric side effects is very long; among the most common offenders are the antihypertensive medications, such as propranolol and reserpine. Propranolol is a β-adrenergic blocking agent that penetrates the CNS, and it is a well-known cause of depression. Reserpine is contained in a number of combination antihypertensive medications. Small dosages (i.e., 0.25 mg daily) can produce severe depression. Levodopa, used in the treatment of Parkinson's disease, can cause behavioral disturbances, including anxiety, hallucinations, and depression, especially in elderly patients. Prednisone, an adrenocorticosteroid, can exaggerate an existing emotional disturbance, including depression. It also can initiate disturbances such as insomnia, psychoses (infrequently), and severe depression. Toxic doses of digoxin may cause delirium with hallucinations, although disorientation and aphasia are more common. Elderly persons are particularly vulnerable to the psychiatric side effects of digoxin, but depression is not a described toxic effect.

7. The answer is E. Lithium can affect the function of several organ systems. It can produce leukocytosis, ECG changes, and hypothyroidism. Although the effect of lithium on the kidneys recently has been disputed, it is generally believed that a renal function test should be performed in persons who will be treated with lithium, since lithium therapy has been associated with impaired urine concentrating ability and with renal interstitial fibrosis. Lithium has little known effect on the liver; thus, liver function testing would be unnecessary in an otherwise healthy person.

8. The answer is B. Bereavement is a very common event in the lives of older people, and uncomplicated bereavement, although a painful phenomenon, is not itself considered a psychiatric disorder. Careful studies of bereaved people have shown that the experience of loss usually begins with a period of emotional numbness and denial, during which the bereaved person is unable to accept the loss. This is followed in days or weeks by a period of longing and yearning and then by mental disorganization. In ideal cases, the bereaved person finally accepts the loss and is able to reconstruct his or her mental and social world without constant mental reference to the dead person. This desirable solution often is unattainable, however.

9. The answer is C. Dementia (organic loss of intellectual function) is the primary cause of significant cognitive impairment among older persons. As the population continues to age, it is anticipated that dementia will become a serious national health issue. Advancing age, apart from concomitant disease, does not lead to cognitive impairment. Cognitive impairment also is not a function of declining intelligence; rather, declining intelligence is a function of dementia. Vitamin deficiency usually is not associated with significant cognitive impairment, although folate or vitamin B_{12} deficiency have been associated with the condition. Depression is a common disorder of the elderly, which mimics dementia in its tendency to cause poor memory and attention span. It is not associated with organic loss of brain function, however.

10. The answer is A. Epidemiologic investigations report that between 2 and 4 million people suffer from irreversible dementias of varying types. The most common irreversible dementia, accounting for more than 50% of all cases, is primary neuronal degeneration associated with Alzheimer's disease. There is progressive deterioration of personality and intelligent behavior ultimately leading to total incapacitation. Learning skills, which are higher cognitive functions, also decline concomitantly with deterioration of personality, intelligent behavior, orientation, and long-term memory. Another important cause of dementia is cerebrovascular disease, probably due to numerous small infarcts. Head trauma, Creutzfeldt-Jakob disease, alcoholism, and Parkinson's disease are less common causes of dementia.

11. The answer is B. A tricyclic antidepressant is an acceptable first choice as an antidepressive agent, particularly for an elderly patient with normal cardiovascular function. Newer "minor" tranquilizers (e.g., benzodiazepines such as alprazolam) sometimes are prescribed for agitated depression; however, they are not licensed by the Food and Drug Administration for this use, and their use in this situation is not established. A β-blocking agent is likely to worsen depression in this patient and should not be used. This patient has a broad spectrum of depressive symptoms, and a sleeping disorder is better managed by treating the underlying illness. The patient has no indications of mania or other psychosis, delirium, or dementia; therefore, neither lithium nor a neuroleptic agent is appropriate.

12. The answer is B. Elderly patients who develop late-onset alcoholism are more likely to have had some form of stress associated with aging, including death of a spouse, retirement, physical illness, or loneliness. Although psychosocial stress is a major contributory factor to late-onset alcoholism, a similar relationship for early-onset alcoholism has not been found. People with a family history of heavy drinking tend to be those with an early, rather than late, onset of alcoholism. Early-onset alcoholics are more likely to have a long history of alcohol-related problems, while late-onset alcoholics either did not drink prior to old age or engaged in sporadic drinking. Only a small percentage of the elderly abuse illicit substances, and those who do generally report a moderate use of alcohol.

13. The answer is A. Lumbar puncture is not a standard procedure for evaluating the cause of significant cognitive impairment. It may be indicated, however, to rule out CNS infection, especially syphilis. A comprehensive evaluation of a patient with significant cognitive impairment may not be performed easily, depending on the person's level of consciousness, motivation, and rapport with the clinician. The evaluation should begin with a careful medical history that includes a drug inventory, followed by a physical examination, neurologic and psychiatric evaluations, and psychological testing for cognitive performance and emotional status. In addition, laboratory procedures should be done, including CBC, folate and vitamin B_{12} levels, serum chemistry screening, erythrocyte sedimentation rate, urinalysis, serology, and thyroid function testing. Radiologic procedures (chest x-ray, brain CT scanning) should be considered in these patients, and an EEG or screening for drug toxicity may be useful.

14. The answer is A. Lithium carbonate is effective in the treatment of the acute phase of mania and as prophylaxis for recurrent episodes. Lithium has a low therapeutic index, however; as a result, lithium treatment often is delayed in the acutely manic patient until sedation is achieved. Treatment of manic elderly patients usually involves initial therapy with antipsychotic medication, which exerts its effects quickly. Because of the possibility of tardive dyskinesia and because antipsychotic medications have not been shown to have any value in the prevention of bipolar disorder, bipolar patients generally are managed after a manic episode with lithium carbonate alone. The prophylactic use of lithium carbonate in the elderly should take into account the various risks associated with lithium use. Because chronic lithium use is associated with conditions such as diffuse goiter, decreased glucose tolerance, interstitial nephritis, thyroid deficiency, and nephrogenic diabetes insipidus, it is advisable not to treat patients with lithium prophylactically unless they have had several prior manic episodes. Although carbamazepine has been used in lithium-resistant patients, it is not recommended for routine prophylaxis for bipolar disorder due to its potentially serious side effects with chronic administration.

15. The answer is C. There are data to support several hypotheses regarding the etiology and pathogenesis of primary neuronal degeneration of the Alzheimer type. Among these hypotheses are cytoarchitectural disruption by intracellular insoluble proteins, neurochemical changes (i.e., cholinergic and noradrenergic system abnormalities), prion infection, and accumulation of exogenous aluminum. Cerebrovascular vasoconstriction is not considered to be a tenable etiologic hypothesis.

16. The answer is B. Defense mechanisms operate to ward off anxiety. They may appear episodically or habitually. Denial, a primitive or infantile defense (i.e., at the lower level of adaptive functioning), has been defined as the disavowing and rejecting of any aspects of internal or external reality that, if acknowledged, would cause anxiety. The patient is denying his obvious drinking problem in spite of the associated physical illness. Thus, he is avoiding the external reality of the cause of his illness. The other defense mechanisms mentioned may play some part in his coping with his alcoholism, but these are not the primary mechanisms used by this alcoholic patient at this time. Projection involves ascribing unacceptable thoughts, feelings, or both to another person. Rationalization constructs acceptable motives for behavior that is unacceptable. In reaction formation, only one, intensified, side of an attitude or relationship is allowed into consciousness (e.g., extreme morality, self-righteousness). Isolation of affect separates a thought from its attached (painful) feeling.

17. The answer is A. In this instance, the patient acknowledges his drinking but disavows his own responsibility and justifies his behavior by attributing it to his wife's nagging. The other defense mechanisms, which fall at the middle to the higher levels of adaptive behavior, do not apply in this situation. Regression is the return to or revival of earlier forms of behavior or thought in response to a current stress. Sublimation takes the energy generated by unacceptable motives or feelings and channels it into socially acceptable behavior.

18. The answer is D. It is expected that the patient would feel sad, frightened, angry, or guilty about having developed cirrhosis from his excessive alcohol consumption. To avoid these uncomfortable feelings, he is using the mechanism of reaction formation to push them out of awareness and claims to be elated about his illness. If the patient were to describe his self-caused serious illness in unemotional terms and claim he felt no anger, sadness, or unhappiness, he would be using the defense of isolation of affect. Counterphobic behavior involves putting oneself in anxiety- or fear-provoking situations as a means of denying that fear exists.

19. The answer is C. Elderly patients, particularly women, are relatively prone to drug-induced parkinsonism (antipsychotic drugs are the predominant offenders), which may present as cogwheel rigidity, bradykinesia, tremor, loss of postural reflexes, masked facies, and drooling. A patient may manifest one, several, or all of these findings, which usually occur in the first few weeks of treatment with one of these drugs. The differential diagnosis is extremely important because an akinetic syndrome easily can be mistaken for a major depressive disorder or an exacerbation of the patient's psychosis in the form of a catatonic stupor. This may be the case, particularly if akinesia is the only prominent parkinsonian feature. The diagnosis usually can be established by careful examination of the patient, which will demonstrate other parkinsonian signs such as cogwheel rigidity and the loss of postural reflexes. A test dose of an antiparkinsonian agent can produce dramatic results if the clinician remains in doubt. There is no hypothyroidism associated with trifluoperazine ingestion. Although patients who are chronically institutionalized may appear apathetic and affectless, these findings should not be confused with those of antipsychotic-induced parkinsonism, as the latter is extremely responsive to specific treatment.

20. The answer is C. The appropriate treatment obviously depends upon the correct diagnosis. Antipsychotic-induced parkinsonian syndrome usually is extremely responsive to an antiparkinsonian agent such as benztropine or trihexyphenidyl. The peripheral and central anticholinergic effects of these agents may produce unwanted side effects themselves, such as blurred vision and urinary retention, which can be particularly troublesome in the elderly. Nevertheless, an antiparkinsonian drug would be the first step in treatment of this patient. An additional approach might be to decrease the dosage of the antipsychotic in question, as resolution of the parkinsonian syndrome sometimes will follow. However, the patient should not be given thyroid hormone unless there is a separate diagnosis of hypothyroidism. A major depressive disorder may follow the resolution of psychotic symptoms in a schizophrenic episode and, if significant, could be treated with an antidepressant along with an antipsychotic. There is no reason to believe that a major depressive episode is the most likely diagnosis in this patient. Increasing the trifluoperazine might be indicated if there has been a clear worsening of the patient's psychosis; however, the clinician must be careful not to mistake neuroleptic catatonia, which is another complication of antipsychotic therapy, for a worsening of the patient's psychosis. Neuroleptic catatonia is treated by discontinuing the antipsychotic therapy. Encouraging the patient to participate in ward activities is a reasonable intervention; however, a patient with untreated akinesia would be unable to respond to such an approach.

21. The answer is A. Some patients may be unable to tolerate high-potency antipsychotics such as trifluoperazine, even with the addition of an antiparkinsonian drug to the regimen. If the patient's psychosis cannot be managed at a lower dosage, a change to a different class of antipsychotics is indicated. Such a patient is likely to do better on one of the lower-potency drugs such as thioridazine or loxapine. Again, the proper treatment depends upon an accurate diagnosis. In the absence of a major depressive episode, neither an antidepressant, a stimulant, nor ECT is indicated. There is no evidence of hypothyroidism, the presence of which would indicate treatment with thyroid hormone.

22. The answer is E. Clinically depressed patients with alcohol problems should generally be given antidepressant medications along with psychotherapy. Sedatives, hypnotics, and tranquilizers are contraindicated if it is known that alcohol is still being abused, even periodically. One-fourth to one-third of patients who are depressed increase their alcohol intake during their depressive bouts. Relieving the depressive state of the patient may lead to reduced alcohol intake as the depressive symptoms improve. Disulfiram is indicated only for impulsive drinkers who wish to stop drinking completely; in this binge drinker, concurrent use of alcohol and disulfiram could cause a serious toxic reaction.

23. The answer is A. Clinically depressed older patients with alcohol problems do very well in group therapy and socialization programs. When combined with antidepressant therapy, attendance at group programs is found to be effective in eliminating alcohol abuse among elderly patients. Efforts at reducing the social and pyschological stresses of aging have also reduced the number of elderly who abuse alcohol. Disulfiram, traditional AA meetings, and intensive alcoholism treatment programs are not as effective with elderly patients as they are with younger alcoholics.

24. The answer is D. The anticholinergic agents found in over-the-counter cold and allergy medications, the antidepressant medication, and periodic alcohol use increase the risk of anticholinergic side effects. The physician must ascertain what possible drug–drug interactions are present and determine the extent of the patient's over-the-counter drug use. Inventory of over-the-counter drug use should be routine in the diagnostic evaluation of all older patients but particularly of those who are known to abuse substances. Although a drug screen may be helpful, it may not reveal the presence of over-the-counter medications. Reducing the dosage of doxepin alone is not sufficient since the drug–drug interaction may still lead to a syndrome of anticholinergic overactivity. Thiamine administration is appropriate for any malnourished alcoholic to prevent thiamine deficiency upon refeeding, but the described syndrome is not one of thiamine deficiency. Bethanechol will not be needed for urinary retention if the anticholinergic side effects can be eliminated.

25–28. The answers are: 25-T, 26-F, 27-T, 28-T. Over-the-counter drug use among the elderly is vastly greater than that among the general population. One study indicated that 69% of people over age 60 use over-the-counter drugs, 40% of them on a daily basis. Increased drug sensitivity due to age promotes the risk of toxicity and dependence. Of all over-the-counter drug users, 80% also use prescribed drugs or alcohol. Because many elderly patients do not disclose the extent of their over-the-counter drug use, physicians (who also neglect to ask) often do not diagnose problems due to these drugs. Over-the-counter drug abusers can be helped by traditional intervention and therapeutic treatment programs for substance abuse.

29–32. The answers are: 29-F, 30-T, 31-F, 32-F. The exact role played by the noradrenergic system in the pathogenesis of Alzheimer's disease is unclear. A reasonable interpretation of the evidence is that aberrations in the cortical noradrenergic system in Alzheimer's disease are likely to be secondary phenomena resulting from severe cholinergic disease and acetylcholine deficiency. Although many researchers have reported that norepinephrine is decreased in Alzheimer's disease, these findings lack sufficient consistency to warrant a final conclusion. Decreased cortical activity of dopamine-β-hydroxylase has been observed in the brains of Alzheimer patients, but these findings are not consistent for every patient. Noradrenergic changes in Alzheimer patients do not correlate with the clinical severity of the disease; using such changes as an indicator of the presence or extent of the disease is far less reliable than using changes in choline acetyltransferase.

33–36. The answers are: 33-T, 34-T, 35-F, 36-T. The rate of suicide remains highest among people who are 65 years of age and older. The greatest number of successful suicides among women occur after the age of 55, although the incidence peaks shortly after menopause. Among men, however, the incidence continues to increase with age, peaking for white men in the ninth decade. Although more suicides are committed by elderly white men, the rate of suicide among older nonwhite men has shown a dramatic increase during the past 10 years and now far exceeds the national rate. Although less likely to express suicidal ideas than younger persons and less likely to attempt suicide, older people are much more likely to complete suicide successfully; they seldom make "gestures." Because of the likelihood that older people will commit suicide without overtly expressing suicidal ideation, a clinician must be particularly vigilant when older patients indicate that they think life is not worth living or when they express that they wish they did not have to live any longer. If suicidal ideas are suspected, a tactful but explicit inquiry is in order.

37–40. The answers are: 37-T, 38-T, 39-T, 40-F. Creutzfeldt-Jakob disease is a rare presenile dementia caused by a prion (subviral protein particle). Several decades separate patients in affected families, which implies a lengthy incubation time. Rapidly evolving dementia, myoclonic seizures, characteristic EEG changes, and quick progression to coma and death are hallmarks of the disease. Neurologic abnormalities associated with Creutzfeldt-Jakob disease begin at an early stage of the disease in a similar fashion to the disease progression observed in dementia of the Alzheimer type. Because of the many clinical variations of Creutzfeldt-Jakob disease and its similarity to Alzheimer's disease, the two are frequently difficult to differentiate.

Surgical transmission of the disease has occurred. The prion is found in CSF, the cornea, the spleen, and other organs. Nonhuman primates have been inoculated, and incubation periods in these animals range from 8 months to several years. The disease is not caused by growth hormone treatment, but a large percentage of recent cases have occurred in patients treated with pooled pituitary extract from presumably infected human brains.

41–44. The answers are: 41-F, 42-T, 43-T, 44-F. Elderly alcoholics generally are more responsive to treatment than their younger counterparts.

Antidepressant medication may be an effective option in patients who use alcohol as a buffer against depression; however, its use must be carefully supervised. Alcohol potentiates the CNS effects of antidepressants. In addition, alcoholics tend to be self-destructive, and the lethal potential of antidepressants is well documented. Although denial does exist in elderly alcoholics, forceful confrontation ordinarily is not necessary, as it is with younger people, to make them realize that they have an alcohol problem.

Disulfiram is prescribed for younger alcoholics but generally is not necessary for the older drinker. When a person being treated with disulfiram ingests even a small amount of alcohol, a major toxic reaction including headache, hypotension, and copious vomiting quickly develops. This reaction could be fatal in an older person. Disulfiram cannot cure alcoholism; its therapeutic use is limited to treatment of chronic alcoholism by behavior modification.

Group and social therapies appear to be more beneficial treatment modalities, especially in elderly populations. Treatment interventions that are socially oriented and that help the elderly alcoholic deal with sociopsychological problems are more appropriate than intensive inpatient rehabilitation programs.

45–48. The answers are: 45-T, 46-T, 47-T, 48-F. Low-potency antipsychotic medications (e.g., thioridazine, chlorpromazine) are commonly prescribed for older demented patients because their sedating effect often is viewed as useful for the agitated, sleepless patient. Certain side effects of these drugs, however, may be confused with the symptoms being treated. The anticholinergic effects may cause an organic hallucinosis, which also may be accompanied by delirium. Restlessness and agitation associated with these medications (akathisia) actually may exceed the agitation of dementia. It is, therefore, necessary to consider carefully the possibility of drug-induced delirium or agitation in demented patients who worsen when given low-potency antipsychotics. Many psychiatrists prefer high-potency drugs as first-line treatment in older demented patients, although these, too, can produce akathisia. Emotional lability is not an established side effect of antipsychotic medications.

49–52. The answers are: 49-T, 50-F, 51-T, 52-T. Up to 30% of people over the age of 60 use laxatives regularly, and 10% abuse them. Overuse of laxatives can lead to metabolic disturbances such as hypokalemia, vitamin deficiencies, and colonic dilation. Phenacetin is the only analgesic definitely associated with analgesic nephropathy. Phenylpropanolamine can cause hypertensive crisis when taken by a person on MAO inhibitor treatment. When used chronically, magnesium-containing antacids can lead to hypermagnesemia, characterized psychologically by confusion. Physical effects include hypotension, sedation, muscle weakness, and ECG changes. Hypercalcemia can also cause confusion, depression, and other psychiatric symptoms.

53–56. The answers are: 53-T, 54-F, 55-T, 56-F. Although it is a significantly less common disorder among older people than major unipolar depression, bipolar disorder is not uncommon in late life. Older bipolar patients usually are people who have suffered from recurrence of mania and depression throughout their lives, although new onset of mania in late life can happen. Because of the nature of bipolar disorder, which often involves lack of judgment, hyperactivity, and hypersexuality, it can be extremely difficult to engage these people in treatment, and they may have to be involuntarily hospitalized. In the geriatric age-group, manic episodes are somewhat atypical, being associated more with agitated depression rather than hyperactivity. Also, manic and depressive characteristics may appear together, causing the person to be angry and irritable. These factors combined with the tendency for manic episodes to be closer together make it particularly difficult to treat elderly patients with bipolar disorder.

57–60. The answers are: 57-F, 58-T, 59-F, 60-T. Anxious or withdrawing patients with hepatic dysfunction present a particular treatment dilemma. If these patients are given too much medication, they become lethargic and sedated; without medication, they often become unmanageable. Several benzodiazepines (most notably diazepam, chlordiazepoxide, and flurazepam) have active metabolites with very long half-lives and, therefore, are inappropriate in a patient with hepatic disease, as the decreased hepatic metabolism would further prolong the effect of these drugs. Liver disease has little effect, however, on the metabolism of either lorazepam or oxazepam, both of which have relatively short half-lives and no active metabolites.

61–64. The answers are: 61-F, 62-F, 63-T, 64-F. Paraphrenia is a commonly seen paranoid disorder characterized by a late-life onset of delusional thinking but no other mental or physical disorder that would explain the delusions. It differs from the delusional syndrome seen in Alzheimer's disease and other dementias in that no cognitive impairment exists. Patients seem well adjusted and even happy in their delusions, which usually are grandiose in nature and well systematized. Confrontation and clarification do little to dispel the unrealistic and implausible character of the delusions. Although sometimes unresponsive to therapeutic intervention, patients with paraphrenic symptoms may respond well to antipsychotic medication. Compliance with a medical regimen, however, is a potential problem in paranoid patients.

Glossary of Abbreviated Terms

AA Alcoholics Anonymous
ACE angiotensin-converting enzyme
ACTH adrenocorticotropic hormone
ADA American Diabetic Association
ADH antidiuretic hormone
AFB acid-fast bacillus
AIDS acquired immune deficiency syndrome
ATPase adenosine triphosphatase
AV node atrioventricular node
B cell B ("bursa-equivalent") lymphocyte
BUN blood urea nitrogen
CBC complete blood cell count
CEA carcinoembryonic antigen
CK creatine kinase
CNS central nervous system
COPD chronic obstructive pulmonary disease
CPPD calcium pyrophosphate dihydrate
CSF cerebrospinal fluid
CT computed tomography
D_2 receptor dopamine$_2$ receptor
DNA deoxyribonucleic acid
DSM-III-R *Diagnostic and Statistical Manual of Mental Disorders*, 3rd ed, revised
DTIC dacarbazine
ECG electrocardiogram
ECT electroconvulsive therapy
EEG electroencephalogram
EMG/NCV studies electromyelography and nerve conduction velocity studies
ER estrogen receptor
FABER maneuver flexion, abduction, and external rotation of the hip
FSH follicle-stimulating hormone
GFR glomerular filtration rate
HCG human chorionic gonadotropin
HLA human leukocyte antigen
HSV-1 herpes simplex virus-1
IgE immunoglobulin E
IgG immunoglobulin G
IgM immunoglobulin M
IVP intravenous pyelography
KUB x-ray flat-plate abdominal (kidney, ureter, and bladder) x-ray
LDH lactate dehydrogenase
LES lower esophageal sphincter
LH luteinizing hormone
LHRH luteinizing hormone-releasing hormone
MAO inhibitors monoamine oxidase inhibitors
MMPI Minnesota Multiphasic Personality Inventory
MPTP synthetic meperidine analogue
MRI magnetic resonance imaging
MSH melanocyte-stimulating hormone
NCAT National Conference on Antithrombotic Therapy
NPH insulin isophane insulin suspension
NSAID nonsteroidal anti-inflammatory drug
PPD purified protein derivative
PT prothrombin time
PTH parathyroid hormone
PTT partial thromboplastin time
S_2 second heart sound
S_3 third heart sound
SA node sinoatrial node
SGOT serum glutamic-oxaloacetic transaminase
SIADH syndrome of inappropriate secretion of antidiuretic hormone
T cell T (thymus-dependent) lymphocyte
T_3 triiodothyronine
T_4 tetraiodothyronine (thyroxine)
TBG thyroxine-binding globulin
TIA transient ischemic attack
TSH thyroid-stimulating hormone
VDRL test Venereal Disease Research Laboratories test

Bibliography

Adams RD, Victor M: *Principles of Neurology*. New York, McGraw-Hill, 1985

Andreoli TE, Carpenter CJ, Plum F, et al (eds): *Cecil Essentials of Medicine*. Philadelphia, WB Saunders, 1986

Andres R, Bierman EL, Hazzard WR (eds): *Principles of Geriatric Medicine*. New York, McGraw-Hill, 1985

Asbury AK, McKhann GM, McDonald WI (eds): *Diseases of the Nervous System*. London, William Heinemann, 1986

Baker AB, Joynt RJ (eds): *Clinical Neurology*, 16th ed. Philadelphia, JB Lippincott, 1984

Ball GV, Koopman WJ (eds): *Clinical Rheumatology*. Philadelphia, WB Saunders, 1986

Beck WW (ed): *Obstetrics and Gynecology*. Media, PA, Harwal/Wiley Medical, 1986

Birren E, Schaie KW (eds): *Handbook of the Psychology of Aging*. New York, Van Nostrand Reinhold, 1985

Branch WT: *Office Practice of Medicine*, 2nd ed. Philadelphia, WB Saunders, 1987

Brocklehurst JC (ed): *Textbook of Geriatric Medicine and Gerontology*, 3rd ed. London, Churchill and Livingstone, 1985

Calkins E, Davis PJ, Ford AB (eds): *The Practice of Geriatrics*. Philadelphia, WB Saunders, 1986

Coakley D (ed): *Acute Geriatric Medicine*. Littleton, MA, PSG Publishing, 1981

Conn HF, Conn RB: *Current Diagnosis No. 7*. Philadelphia, WB Saunders, 1984

Covington TR, Walker JI (eds): *Current Geriatric Therapy*. Philadelphia, WB Saunders, 1984

Cummings JL, Benson DF: *Dementia: A Clinical Approach*. Boston, Butterworths, 1983

Dalen JE, Hirsch J (eds): American College of Chest Physicians and National Heart, Lung, and Blood Institute National Conference on Antithrombotic Therapy. *Chest* 89:2(Suppl), 1986

Delafuente JC, Stewart RB: *Therapeutics in the Elderly*. Baltimore, Williams & Wilkins, 1988

DeVita VT, Hellman S, Rosenberg, SA (eds): *Cancer: Principles & Practice of Oncology*, 2nd ed. Philadelphia, JB Lippincott, 1985

Gilman AG, Goodman LS, Rall TW, et al (eds): *The Pharmacological Basis of Therapeutics*, 7th ed. New York, Macmillan Publishing, 1985

Ham RJ (ed): *Geriatric Medicine Annual*. Kansas City, MO, Society for Teachers of Family Medicine, 1986

Hansten PD: *Drug Interactions: Clinical Significance of Drug–Drug Interactions*, 5th ed. Philadelphia, Lea & Febiger, 1985

Hurst JW, Rackley C (eds): *Medicine for the Practicing Physician*, 6th ed. New York, McGraw-Hill, 1985

Jacob LS (ed): *Pharmacology*, 2nd ed. Media, PA, Harwal/Wiley Medical, 1987

Jarrell BE, Carabasi RA (eds): *Surgery*. Media, PA, Harwal/Wiley Medical, 1986

Jefferson JW, et al (eds): *Lithium Encyclopedia for Clinical Practice*. Washington, DC, Psychiatric Press, 1987

Jenike MA: *Handbook of Geriatric Psychopharmacology*, Littleton, MA, PSG Publishing, 1985

Katcher B, Young L, Koda-Kimble M: *Applied Therapeutics*, 3rd ed. Spokane, WA, Applied Therapeutics, 1983

Kelley WN, Harris ED, Ruddy S, et al (eds): *Textbook of Rheumatology*, 2nd ed. Philadelphia, WB Saunders, 1985

McEvoy GK, McQuarrie GM (eds): *Drug Information '87*. Bethesda, MD, American Society of Hospital Pharmacists, 1987

Mazzaferri EL: *Endocrinology Case Studies*, 3rd ed. New York, Medical Examination Publishing, 1986

Messeri F: *Current Clinical Practice*. Philadelphia, WB Saunders, 1987

Myers AR (ed): *Medicine*. Media, PA, Harwal/Wiley Medical, 1986

Pathy MSJ (ed): *Principles and Practice of Geriatric Medicine*. New York, John Wiley, 1985

Petersdorf R, Adams RD, Braunwald E, et al (eds): *Harrison's Principles of Internal Medicine*, 10th ed. New York, McGraw-Hill, 1983

Rakel RR (ed): *Conn's Current Therapy*. Philadelphia, WB Saunders, 1986

Reichel W (ed): *Clinical Aspects of Aging*, 2nd ed. Baltimore, Williams & Wilkins, 1983

Rossman I (ed): *Clinical Geriatrics*, 3rd ed. Philadelphia, JB Lippincott, 1986

Rubenstein E, Federman DD (eds): *Scientific American: Medicine*. New York, Scientific American, 1987

Scully JH (ed): *Psychiatry*. Media, PA, Harwal/Wiley Medical, 1985

Simonson W: *Medications and the Elderly: A Guide for Promoting Proper Use*. Rockville, MD, Aspen, 1984

Sleisenger MH, Fordtran JS (eds): *Gastrointestinal Disease*, 4th ed. Philadelphia, WB Saunders, 1988

Vinken PJ, Bruyn GW (eds): *Handbook of Clinical Neurology*, vol. 49. New York, Elsevier Scientific, 1986

Walshe TM (ed): *Manual of Clinical Problems in Geriatric Medicine*. Boston, Little, Brown, 1985

Walton J (ed): *Brain's Diseases of the Nervous System*, 9th ed. Oxford, Oxford University Press, 1985

Wells C (ed): *Dementia*. Philadelphia, Davis, 1977

Wiener JM (ed): *Behavioral Science*. Media, PA, Harwal/Wiley Medical, 1987

Wintrobe MM, Lee GR, Boggs DR, et al (eds): *Clinical Hematology*, 8th ed. Philadelphia, Lea & Febiger, 1981

Wyngaarden JB, Smith LH (eds): *Cecil Textbook of Medicine*, 18th ed. Philadelphia, WB Saunders, 1988

Zarit S: *Aging and Mental Disorders: Psychological Approaches to Assessment and Treatment*, New York, Free Press, 1983